Alison's journey to good health should be an in
challenged every modern-day paradigm and explored all possible
must be one of the most complex and least understood diseases of the 21st century. It
is rare to see such a spectrum of therapies and concepts discussed in one book.
Detailed explanations of human physiology sit comfortably alongside eloquent descriptions of how energy and emotions affect our health.

Alison has set out to leave no stone unturned in her quest to produce what will
become the definitive guide for sufferers of chronic fatigue.

Alessandro Ferretti, Dip ION, mBANT
Lecturer and clinical nutritionist

This book is for anyone who wants to feel better. Drawing upon the knowledge she
gained in resolving her own health issues, Dr Adams, in an informative and understandable fashion, gives the fundamental and underlying causes of most disease. She
then gives you the tools and information you need to tackle your own health problems.

Dr Mark Breiner, DDS, FAGD, FIAOMT
US holistic dentist and author of *Whole Body Dentistry*

A tour de force – comprehensive, well researched and well written. An extraordinary
self-help guide.

Jane Thurnell-Read, MSc, KF Fellow
Kinesiologist and author of *Allergy A to Z*, *Geopathic Stress* and other books

A very comprehensive and important guide for both sufferers and practitioners. As a
practising mercury-free dentist, I can confirm that the release of mercury from dental
amalgam is one of the biggest underestimated factors affecting general health today.

Peter Mendelsohn, BDS (Sydney)

This is an impressive book because it argues from experience and will be of great help to people who have had these problems without being able to find help. This book charts new thinking in this important subject.

M E Clarke, BA, BSc
Nutritionist

This is an extremely well written and informative book that deserves to be read not only by fatigue sufferers, but also by natural health practitioners. Understanding the cause is the first step to recovery. This book will bring hope to those suffering with chronic fatigue syndrome.

Lesley Sarson, KF (Assoc)
Complementary health practitioner

Chronic Fatigue, ME, and Fibromyalgia: The Natural Recovery Plan

Alison Adams

BDS (Lond.), MS (Michigan), KFRP,
Dip I K, Dip Class K, MRAT,
H I Dip (Complementary Therapies),
Dip Life Coaching, Dip Past Life Therapy

WATKINS PUBLISHING

LONDON

Distributed in the USA and Canada by Sterling Publishing Co., Inc.
387 Park Avenue South, New York, NY 10016–8810

This edition first published in the UK and USA 2010 by
Watkins Publishing, Sixth Floor, Castle House,
75–76 Wells Street, London W1T 3QH

1 3 5 7 9 10 8 6 4 2

Designed by Jerry Goldie Graphic Design
Typeset by Dorchester Typesetting Group

Printed and bound in Great Britain

Library of Congress Cataloging-in-Publication Data Available

ISBN: 978-1-906787-76-9

www.watkinspublishing.co.uk
For information about custom editions, special sales, premium
and corporate purchases, please contact Sterling Special Sales
Department at 800-805-5489 or specialsales@sterlingpub.com

Contents

List of Illustrations

Disclaimer

The information in this book is provided for informational purposes only and is not intended as a substitute for professional medical advice, diagnosis or treatment. If you are suffering from any medical conditions or health problems, it is recommended that you consult the appropriate medical professional. If you are pregnant, trying to become pregnant or are breastfeeding it is expressly recommended that you *do not undertake any detoxification* including that outlined in this book. The protocol suggested in this book is intended for adults and is not suitable for children, for whom appropriate professional advice should be sought.

Neither the publishers, the author, nor others associated with this work accept liability or responsibility for any person or entity for any loss or damage caused or claimed to have been caused directly or indirectly by or from the information or ideas contained, suggested or referenced in this book or from any errors, misstatements, inaccuracies or omissions in the content whether inadvertent or not, that may be found in the text. Every individual is unique and no method of treatment is effective for everyone. You are strongly encouraged to become informed and take responsibility for your own health-care decisions based upon your research and in partnership with a qualified health-care professional and neither the author nor publishers accept liability for readers who self-prescribe. All supplements should be kept out of the reach of infants and small children.

This book is dedicated to my husband Mark,
who made it possible by supporting me financially and emotionally
and who never doubted that I was gravely ill.

I extend this dedication to all those who have suffered throughout
history – and who continue to suffer at the hands of the medical
and dental professions.

Acknowledgements

I wish to acknowledge all those on whose shoulders I stand, many of whom have been pilloried and worse, but who chose to stick their heads above the parapet because it was the right thing to do. I also wish to recognize the efforts of the many committed natural therapists over the years who have toiled away often without much recognition or reward. I would particularly like to thank the developer of kinesiology, Dr George Goodheart, who left the world an incredible tool with which to understand health and disease. Some people know that they have touched your life, but a great many others do not. Of those who are possibly unaware of their impact I would especially like to acknowledge the work of Dr Dietrich Klinghardt, Dr Hal Huggins and Louise Hay. Of those that are aware of their role in my life I would like to thank all my many teachers over the years including Jackie Norton and Pauline Noakes for their wisdom, experience and patience. Finally, I would like to especially thank Vicki Edgson for writing the Foreword, Dr Mark Breiner, Dr Peter Mendelsohn, Jane Thurnell-Read, M E Clarke, Lesley Sarson and Alessandro Ferretti for their endorsements, and Dr Dietrich Klinghardt for permitting the use of figure 6.

> **Never doubt that a small group of thoughtful, committed citizens can change the world. Indeed, it is the only thing that ever has.**
>
> **Margaret Mead**

Foreword

Firstly, for anyone who has suffered from any form of long-term illness, and been through the desperation and indignation of not 'being heard', you will recognize, in this superb book, compassion from a fellow-sufferer that goes way beyond her practitioner experience. Alison's personal experience draws you in from the first page, and persuades you to follow her every painstaking step of the way, to a road of recovery.

Furthermore, for those who have been unfortunate enough to fall down any one of the myriad routes that lead to chronic fatigue syndrome, fibromyalgia, post-traumatic stress syndrome, or others, such a recovery is not easy – it flies in the face of the opinions of every medical practitioner you may have come across to date, every tried and trusted professional and specialist, even your own GP (especially your own GP, as he/she may well have referred you to many of the professionals whose waiting rooms you have sat in nervously, anxiously praying for an 'answer' to your problems). But even more challenging will be the barrage of disrespect for your decision to 'take the alternative route' as absurd, risky, inconsiderate and potentially life-threatening, by the very people for whom your recovery should be so important. As one of those 'alternative practitioners' myself, I would urge you to follow your instinct, as Alison did, despite all the professional knowledge on offer, and start to enquire about some of the other remedial techniques on offer that can allow your body to start to heal itself.

The first principle of naturopathic medicine is 'Do no Harm', as the author so rightly points out – appreciating that your body is the most incredibly complex and sophisticated collection of organs that were designed to interact with each other on a moment-to-moment basis of ultimate survival. What has happened on your journey may not be the same as Alison Adams', or mine, but the result is the same – confusion and intoxication of the very systems in your body that were designed to work synergistically for your survival. Undoing the harm that has occurred by removing many of those self-imposed toxins (as well as some that you were not aware of in your surroundings) is the first step in responsibility that you can take for yourself. But first you need a guide (or several!) to show you exactly what may have intoxicated your body, and how you might start unravelling the damage. In doing this, you will be 'talking to your body' and letting it know that you are willing to help it to help you.

The extraordinary fact about this book is that it is written by a woman who had trained in the allopathic practice of dentistry, which seems straightforward enough in itself. However, her own experience with rapidly deteriorating health forced her (at a risk to her own most personal relationships and colleague respect) to question the very nature of allopathic medicine, medications and the very approaches in which she had so diligently trained – ultimately to reject them all. Not easy within the medical profession – and especially when she was already 'worn down' by her own illness.

What strikes me most is how Alison's innate sense of survival has driven her to look into all possibilities within the complementary health field, not at a superficial level, but ultimately to study each topic that she found to be affecting her adversely, that she might assure herself of being 'properly equipped' to address each of the causes of her own physical breakdown. That she has undertaken to subsequently share these studies, along with the research of many other masters within their field, and bring all together in this book is nothing less than a gift that should not be spurned.

The beauty of this book is that Alison has sought out the best practices and remedies, explaining in great detail why, when and how to employ them. It may not be easy initially to take on board the enormity of the dedication, cost or challenges that face you in your recovery programme but, if you make the commitment to read the book in the first place, you will find therein a wealth of knowledge, research and answers that you may not have had the energy to undertake yourself without specific guidance and reassurance. Once equipped with such knowledge, you will then be in a better, stronger place to seek out the necessary guides to help you on your road to recovery.

I feel honoured to have been asked to write a foreword for this excellent book, and humbled by the degree of professional enquiry and research with which Alison has approached this massive topic for which allopathic medicine still has no answer, other than 'plenty of rest'. When my own niece was diagnosed with 'chronic fatigue syndrome' following a bout of 'typical teenage glandular fever' last year, my heart sank that I would be able to do little to help her, as my history of practising the 'complementary therapies' has taught me to stand back from my own family and close friends, unless asked to participate, particularly when they are fearful of the outcome. In my own practice, I frequently have patients who consult me when they are literally at the end of their tether, too exhausted to try any further treatments.

Alison, I salute you for this excellent book – as a fellow practitioner, I applaud your passion, tenacity and unerring dedication to share with others what you have undertaken so painfully for your own health, and painstakingly researched and recorded for others to benefit from. This book is a gift to both patients and practitioners alike, as I know that anyone who reads it will also testify. I would have been proud to have written such a book myself!

To the reader – find a quiet place, give yourself the time you so desperately need, and turn over the page to begin your own road to recovery!

Vicki Edgson, Dip ION
Nutritionist and naturopath, author and television presenter

Introduction

Fifty per cent of what you have been taught is wrong.
The trouble is – you don't know which fifty per cent.

Axiom

I come from a family with an extensive history of autoimmune disorders; many of my female relatives have died of their illnesses comparatively young after enduring a lifetime of low-grade health. I, too, had experienced a lifetime of multiple chronic health problems and the associated pharmaceutical, surgical and physical interventions before eventually degenerating into a health crisis in mid-life. Over the years I had also consulted many different complementary practitioners, all of whose initial confidence that their therapy would help ultimately proved unfounded. Professionally, my enquiring mind managed to survive formal education, a UK Bachelor's and a US Master's degree in dentistry and twenty years of dental practice. I remember that, even when being taught the conventional medical model at dental school it was obvious to me that there were large, important and frustrating pieces of the jigsaw puzzle missing. When I eventually became desperately ill it took me far too long to realize that the medical profession not only would not but, I now understand, could not help me. This was shocking to me at the time, but in retrospect I am grateful for it because this was the moment when I determined that since I wasn't ready to follow my relatives to an early grave, I would have to figure out the answers for myself.

I sold my dental practice and, over time, I found people and therapies that did help. I eventually retrained in various different aspects of natural health including kinesiology (a way of 'talking' to the body in a language it understands using muscle testing to determine the responses) and allergy therapy. Although I was fairly open-minded and, more importantly, desperate, this required leaving the shores of certainty behind in search of a new conceptual territory and was very confronting. Like the optical-illusion picture of the beautiful young girl and the old crone with which you are probably familiar, there is more than one way of looking at health and illness – and this time all the pieces of the jigsaw puzzle fit together. The central tenet of naturopathy is to identify, treat and remove the cause of illness rather than treating the symptoms as most often happens.

Using a particular technique to uncover hidden toxins, I became convinced that occult mercury toxicity is playing a huge causative role in most of the illnesses that we are witnessing in the developed world. Effectively, sufferers of chronic fatigue syndrome, fibromyalgia and autoimmune diseases are acting as the 'canaries in the mine' of our current way of living – they are the vulnerable ones in a society whose members will all inevitably follow in their footsteps. For obvious reasons, this was not an easy or comfortable discovery for me. For my own part, I had been subjected to the mercury preservative in all the usual vaccinations, had a not-inconsiderable number of amalgam fillings, twenty-five years of occupational exposure and finally – and nearly fatally – an accidental spill of an amalgam cartridge in one of my surgeries that was never located. In retrospect, I could clearly see how each of these events had been another nail in my coffin.

My goal in writing *Chronic Fatigue, ME and Fibromyalgia: The Natural Recovery Plan* was to produce the book that I needed and could not find when I was ill. Whilst I appreciate that there are many dedicated specialists with an interest in this topic, it turns out that there is no greater motivator than having your life depend upon finding the solutions! In this book I present the answers that I found and I have incorporated my knowledge as a dentist, holistic therapist and former sufferer. Chronic fatigue syndrome, ME, fibromyalgia and autoimmune disorders are, in fact, slightly different manifestations of the same problem and share root causes and so will be referred to collectively throughout this book as fatigue-related syndromes or FRS. The information in this book is organized into two sections. Part 1 addresses the various factors contributing to fatigue-related syndromes and Part 2 examines the various elements involved in recovery. Some of the information may appear rather unnecessary or irrelevant to your current predicament, but please try to at least grasp a flavour of what is being communicated. Throughout the book some fairly technical detail has been included and you may choose to skip or scan this information. In any event, whether you understand or accept some of the material presented is less important than implementing the solutions set out in the second part of this book.

I hope to spare you the decades of expense and suffering that I endured and the necessity of abandoning your career in order to retrain as a naturopath! My deepest wish is that the information in this book helps to guide you most efficiently out of the quicksands of CFS and fibromyalgia. However, a bit like the mythical yokel being asked directions and replying, 'You don't want to start from here,' you are most probably going to need to let go of everything that you think you know about these illnesses and, more generally, about health and disease, and then we can truly begin.

Part 1

The Problems

Problems are messages.

Shakti Gawain

Give nonsense a good head-start with Tradition and Habit cheering it from the sidelines, and if you think Reform can catch up with it inside of two or three thousand years or more, your opinion is contrary to experience.

Author unknown

There are three classes of people: Those who see. Those who see when they are shown. Those who do not see.

Leonardo Da Vinci

Chapter 1
'Here Be Dragons'

When you seek a new path to truth, you must expect
to find it blocked by expert opinion.

Albert Guerard

The chances are that you are reading this book because you believe yourself to have chronic fatigue, ME, fibromyalgia or a similar fatigue-related syndrome and the solutions that have been offered so far aren't working. Alternatively, you may be managing your illness using pharmaceuticals and wish to find a better or more permanent solution.

You have probably trusted health professionals you perceive to be powerful and knowledgeable with your precious health up to this point and, as we shall see, this is a big part of the problem. Frankly, many (if not most) doctors don't believe in the existence of FRS and those that do don't know what has caused it or how to treat it. So how can you expect them to help you, when they don't understand what is wrong? Considerable and indeed total recovery from FRS is entirely possible, but much of your ability to recover lies in your own hands and may present the biggest challenge of your life to date. Your journey back to health starts with the total rejection of the most likely probable outcomes: either to remain at your current level of debility or to become more degeneratively ill and possibly die prematurely. Next is the absolute determination that nothing less than full recovery and a full life is an acceptable goal. When you commit to doing whatever is necessary to become whole and healthy, you have taken the first and most important step on your new healing path.

Fatigue-Related Syndromes

Fatigue-related syndromes are a complex problem with a multifaceted solution and recovery is probably going to require a fundamental shift in your current view of illness, and possibly of reality. They graphically illustrate a fault line in our commonly accepted beliefs about health and illness and exist in an uncharted territory outside of current orthodox medical thinking in the same way that ancient maps marked the unexplored with 'Here be dragons'. You may find that a lot of your preconceived ideas need to be challenged in order to heal and to believe in the possibility of total healing and this may be very confronting.

The Causes of FRS

Most books describe chronic fatigue syndrome and fibromyalgia as being multifactorial and offer fairly non-specific solutions. Although FRS is multifactorial, three causative factors stand head and shoulders above the rest and, if addressed, result in recovery for most sufferers. The most significant factor is metal toxicity in general and mercury toxicity (mostly from amalgam fillings) in particular, and this is addressed in detail in chapter 9. The other causative factors are viral and other infections, and stress and trauma which are examined in chapters 8 and 11 respectively.

The proposed mechanism is that whilst we are all exposed to toxins the whole time, when we are traumatized or stressed the normal paths of excretion are temporarily suspended, resulting in the accumulation of toxins in specific tissues according to the emotions being experienced. These toxins are then absorbed into the nerves that control the automatic functions in these organs and slowly track up these nerves into the brain and central nervous system. As the tissues become toxic, various viruses and fungi are able to prosper and, finally, parasites may be able to grow unchallenged by the disabled immune system as shown in figure 1.

The good news is that these causes are eminently treatable. The bad news is that

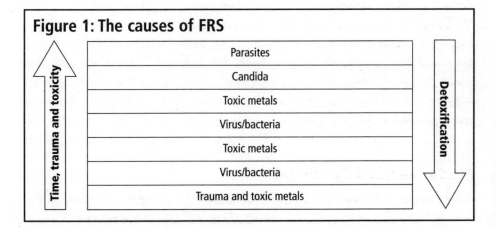

Figure 1: The causes of FRS

Time, trauma and toxicity

| Parasites |
| Candida |
| Toxic metals |
| Virus/bacteria |
| Toxic metals |
| Virus/bacteria |
| Trauma and toxic metals |

Detoxification

effective treatment is going to cost at least as much as an average automobile, is probably going to take several years and requires a lot of commitment and effort. Whilst I have speculated as to mechanisms by which the illness produces so many diverse symptoms, I am confident that the primary causative factors identified are valid. I make this statement based upon the successful outcomes achieved by myself and other practitioners addressing these factors, my own personal experience and because, speaking as a kinesiologist, the same causative factors occur not only in all FRS sufferers, but in most serious and chronic illness. For this reason, whilst this book is primarily intended for those suffering with FRS, the strategies suggested can be applied to most degenerative and chronic illnesses and especially autoimmune diseases. If you know someone who is serious about recovery, irrespective of their condition, please recommend to them the approach outlined in this book. Also, as with everything in life, the problem is infinitely more complex to remedy than it would have been to prevent so please inform others about the causes enumerated in this book to prevent them falling into the same hole you are in.

The Future of Health Care

The ultimate irony is that most of us have willingly submitted to this toxic overload of our systems by having vaccinations, taking pharmaceuticals – many preventatively – and undergoing dental work. Those who contributed to the toxic assault were, by and large, well-intentioned people who thought that they were doing the right thing. Indeed, I can feel no anger because as a dentist I, too, was one of those people. Knowing what I now know, I feel a great deal of guilt about the harm I may have unwittingly done to others and with the best of motives – even to my nearest and dearest. My dental patients trusted me and I trusted the powers-that-be, and we were both misguided and ill-informed.

My hope is that in the very near future, when the new intake of medical and dental students is taught about the recent history of their professions, they will regard many of our 'modern' practices with the incredulity they deserve. The use of mercury – the most potent neurotoxin known to man – in dental amalgam is a 19th-century technology that we are still using in the 21st century. Putting aside concerns about toxins, people are not keen to have ugly corroded silver fillings in their mouth. I also hope that the young medical students will question the need to preventatively inject infective material into healthy subjects under the guise of the vaccination programme.

Recovering from FRS

In his book *Love, Medicine and Miracles*, the surgeon Dr Bernie Siegel describes the characteristics of the small minority of cancer patients who either recovered or outlived all reasonable expectations for survival. He found that whilst they understood the prognosis on offer, they all took complete responsibility for their lives and their health and made all the changes necessary to support their healing. You too need to become your own counsel and expert; after all, you are the world authority on you. No one else, no matter how dedicated, is ever going to be as interested in your health as you are. Ultimately, the journey to happiness and health is one that you undertake for yourself and by yourself and whilst others can assist you along the way, no one else can do it for you – you have to do it yourself.

Your body is going to be your greatest ally in recovery and if you haven't always treated it with the respect that it deserves, then now is a good time to start. The changes that you are going to need to make are outlined in Part 2 and include adopting a diet and supplement regime that supports your body's routes of elimination (chapters 14 and 17 respectively) and addressing some old emotional wounds (chapter 15). You will also need to reduce your future exposure to some commonly occurring toxins (chapter 13) and possibly have some dental work done to remove an ongoing source of toxicity (chapter 18).

You will need to prioritize getting well financially too. In purely monetary terms, what is the point in having holidays, nice clothes or a good car if you are ill? Sell your car and get a cheaper one. Give up alcohol, new clothes, dining out, holidays, smoking or buying a newspaper every day. Find the money. Hopefully, you will recover and be able to earn and enjoy lots more money in the decades to come.

> **The more serious the illness, the more important it is for you to fight back, mobilizing all your resources – spiritual, emotional, intellectual, physical.**
>
> **Norman Cousins**

The Strangest Gift

This may be hard for you to comprehend right now, but life has a funny way of presenting your greatest opportunity as your biggest problem and in time you may even be grateful for your illness. Appreciate that your body has done the least damaging thing at all times in spite of being confronted with an overwhelming assault of toxins and that its actions to date have kept you alive. It may only be half a life, but you are still here to tell the tale. As terrible as I felt when I was ill, other friends and colleagues passed away suddenly or tragically during my fight for health. Ultimately, I was glad that I had been given the time and opportunity to recover. However, in the early days my biggest fear was that my fatigue-related syndrome *wouldn't* actually kill me and that I would be left with a fraction of a life for the rest of my days. Our illnesses are our greatest teachers and the greatest test of our strength. You will certainly not emerge from this experience the same person you were before, but something good invariably comes from testing circumstances if you allow it to, and if you look with the right eyes. Recovering from a fatigue-related syndrome has been by far the toughest challenge of my life and it may be of yours too. My wish for you is that you find the wind beneath your wings and the grit in your soul on your journey.

Chapter 2
We Are Here

Truth is whatever is subjectively convincing given your
current state of consciousness.

David R Hawkins, MD, PhD

We are constantly encouraged to marvel at the sophistication of our technologies and the latest innovations in pharmaceutical solutions and we look back in disbelief at the technologies of yesterday. History, it seems, has taught us nothing. Victorian medicine, in its day, commanded great respect for its practitioners who were probably proud of their 'modern' techniques involving preparations of mercury, arsenic, iron and phosphorous, prescriptions for bleeding and the use of leeches. We now wonder why we embraced the use of DDT fertilizer, asbestos in buildings and the x-raying of children's feet in shoe shops quite so unquestioningly. We are, of course, currently – knowingly or unknowingly – committing similar mistakes on a monumental scale and you are most probably an innocent victim. The problem is that the answers are hidden in plain view, but are invisible to many because of our entire approach to both science and medicine. It is to these two subjects that we now turn our attention.

The Problem with Science

The way science is currently funded and evaluated, we are learning more
and more about less and less, and science has become our enemy instead of
our friend.

Dr Robert Becker

At any given time we are working on the basis of what we currently believe to be the case and we build a paradigm which explains our understanding. We formulate theories and devise experiments where we gather objective and reproducible data to either support or refute our theory. Anecdotal evidence and results that were documented but that are not reproducible are dismissed. However, when a lot of observations fall outside of the boundaries of the current paradigm, a dilemma presents itself. Some remain attached to the existing paradigm by dismissing all the information that does not fit their model. Alternatively, this 'inconvenient' data can indicate the need for a new paradigm that encompasses all the known information. This is what happened with the leap between Newton's solid and material model of the world and Einstein's breakthrough understanding in quantum physics. Remember that once all the greatest minds believed the Earth was flat and vociferously resisted the shocking concept of the planet being a sphere. These shifts are dramatic and hard to accept for those wedded to the contemporary concepts.

When our current paradigm cannot explain certain phenomena, scientists confidently assure us that the paradigm is sound and that it is only a matter of time until science will be able to explain the anomalous data. This is known as promissory materialism and ultimately requires an unscientific act of blind faith. We all resist change, although it is the one inevitability. It is said that no one ever really changes their mind, it is just that those adhering to the old paradigm die and are replaced by others schooled in the new paradigm. In fact, this goes even deeper. We all see the world through filters whereby only a tiny amount of the data available to the unconscious is ever brought to the attention of the conscious mind. So what you are not consciously made aware of, for you, simply does not exist. This is an incredibly powerful process that determines your experience of reality. Also, according to our unfolding understanding of quantum physics, consciousness and matter are interactive, with matter appearing to change from the potential of a wave into particles which organize themselves to conform to our expectations when observed. This means that there is no such thing as a truly objective observation, only participation with an interactive universe, and so the researcher's expectations will inevitably colour the outcome of any study.

> **Every person takes the limits of their own field of vision for the limits of the world.**
>
> **Arthur Schopenhauer**

Sometimes scientists arrogantly claim that our current scientific understanding can explain everything. Well, it is just not true. The more we investigate some things, the more unfathomable they become. For instance, many believed that mapping the human genome would provide definitive answers when, in fact, the project has raised many more questions than it answered. Another troubling matter is that we cannot currently account for most of our universe which we conveniently ascribe to dark energy or dark matter. We cannot even explain gravity or the properties of water, for goodness' sake! Where do thoughts come from? Can you measure love? Where does the mind reside? How are memories stored? These are interesting questions to which our current answers seem woefully inadequate.

Our senses actually inform us about only a tiny amount of the entire electromagnetic spectrum. As such, the very notions of gamma rays, holograms, lasers and sonic scanning would have seemed fanciful to our great grandparents. We are always limited by the technologies of the time and whilst we have now developed equipment that can generate and detect these wavelengths, to imagine that this might be the final word on the matter would prove foolish in the extreme. Science appears to insist that anything that cannot currently be measured does not exist. However, contemporary technologies such as Kirlian photography and Polycontrast Interference Photography (PIP) are now capturing a world of subtle energies previously ignored or unexplored by science.

Finally, science has always worked on the basis of studying the parts in order to explain the whole. The scientific methods of dissection, preparing slides of dead material and using colliders to split the atom are all symptomatic of this way of thinking. The problem with this approach is that, to paraphrase the author Douglas Adams, if you take a cat apart to see how it works, what you have is a non-working cat. Whilst the information gained in this way is undoubtedly useful, it can never provide a complete explanation of observations and certainly not in any kind of larger context.

Finally, there are the technical issues of how studies were set up, what measures were taken, what statistical analysis was performed and how findings were interpreted. This is in addition to any (probably) unintentional researcher bias and funding issues. Researchers make their findings public to interested parties by publishing in refereed journals. This means that other experts (peers) in the field review your paper before publication and this makes it harder to publish any research that contradicts the currently held theory *du jour* than it is to publish confirmatory research. Unfavourable or contradictory findings and experiments that show no association between the factors being studied often never see the light of day, and yet it is still important to share this information with the scientific community. There are also the very human unseen influences of allegiances, political expedience, rivalries, egos and so on which cannot be ignored.

The Problem with 'Conventional' Medicine

First, do no harm.

Hippocrates

It is unclear exactly how 'conventional' medicine earned that epithet since Traditional Chinese Medicine, for instance, is believed by some to have been around for 12,000 years and 'conventional' medicine probably only for the last century or so! For this reason conventional or orthodox medicine will be referred to as allopathic medicine in this book. Whilst both allopathic and holistic medicine agree that all disease is the end result of either genetic abnormalities, infection, radiation, chemical or physical injury and/or trauma and degeneration, the agreement ends there. The approach to, and relative importance of these factors creates a division that is hard to breach. The two main thrusts of allopathic treatment are either to remove the offending body part (usually surgically) or to 'block' the symptoms of disease chemically using pharmaceuticals. This dominant allopathic view is also imposed by law in many instances. Compulsory vaccination programmes, compulsory medicalized childbirth in some states and the widespread illegality of treating cancer using any means other than the allopathic approach (which has woeful results) are all examples. Health insurance, too, often only recognizes and funds allopathic treatments. First, we will address some of the problems inherent in the surgical and pharmaceutical approaches and then some of the wider problems with allopathic medicine.

In all affairs it's a healthy thing now and then to hang a question mark on the things you have long taken for granted.

Bertrand Russell

The Trouble with Surgery

There is no doubt that surgery is a necessary evil at times. However, it is traumatic, unpleasant and painful and it is quite a big challenge for an already sick person to recover from major surgery. It is also avoidable much of the time, if more effective treatment had been undertaken sooner. Even our surgical solutions do not always deliver the benefits hoped for and can create other complications such as adhesions and scar tissue. We all know of people who have had surgery only to have a relapse or recurrence, or who then develop another serious illness. These facts are not unrelated, for reasons that hopefully will become clear.

The Trouble with Drugs

Until the 1920s, all medicine had been naturopathic (natural) and the doctors of the time only had a handful of drugs at their disposal. Within ninety years the pharmaceutical industry has grown from these modest beginnings to become one of the biggest and most profitable industries in the world. Annual global sales currently approach $3 trillion (over £2 trillion) and this owes a great deal to the intervention of two billionaires. A century ago John D Rockefeller and Andrew Carnegie sought to invest their wealth in the emerging pharmaceutical industry. By controlling funding they succeeded in having all the medical schools in the USA that did not exclusively promote the pharmaceutical approach closed down. Half of this behemoth's custom is now currently in the USA with five billion prescriptions being filled each year. Europe comes in a poor second and the developing world represents a rapidly growing market.

The medical profession and the pharmaceutical industry have now become so mutually interdependent that many regard the relationship as being unhealthy and not necessarily operated in the highest interests of patients. Healthcare has effectively become the illness business. In fact, even Dr Halfdan Mahler, a former Director General of the World Health Organization, stated in 1984, 'The major and most expensive part of medical knowledge as applied today appears to be operated more for the satisfaction of the health professions than for the benefit of the consumers of health care'. Doctors write the prescriptions for the drugs and so the pharmaceutical companies compete to influence the doctors. The pharmaceutical companies employ some pretty sharp business practices and relentless lobbying to both protect and expand their market share, as is modern business practice. By some reckonings, there are nearly as many pharmaceutical representatives as doctors in the USA and over 100,000 pharmaceutical lobbyists relentlessly making representations to members of Congress. Finally, slick marketing and advertising campaigns mean that we are collectively held in thrall to the promise the pharmaceutical approach appears to offer.

> **It is difficult to get a man to understand something when his job depends on not understanding it.**
>
> **Upton Sinclair**

The 'Triumphs' of Modern Medicine

It is often touted that modern medicine has 'cured' many diseases, but let's look at that claim a little more closely.

- Nearly half the population of developed countries suffers with at least one chronic ailment.

- Depression, anxiety and ADHD have reached epidemic proportions. To quote Bruce Charlton, 'Mental health and well-being are so rare as to be remarkable,' and 'Psychiatric impairment is the norm.'
- If we survive childhood, our average life expectancy is only *three years longer* than it was a century ago and our total life span has remained static and may be decreasing. Whilst there may be more years in our life, there may not be more life in our years. We are not really living longer – we are just taking longer to die.
- Adverse reactions to properly prescribed pharmaceuticals kill more than 10,000 people each year in the UK and more than 100,000 a year in the USA. This costs the NHS in the UK nearly half a billion pounds a year.
- Pharmaceuticals are, by definition, toxic – they have to be to get a licence! The 'safe' dose is calculated from the lethal dose, which kills 50 per cent of the laboratory rats (LD50).
- All pharmaceuticals work by *suppressing symptoms temporarily* and all pharmaceuticals have unwanted side effects that are often mistaken for other conditions and treated with … more pharmaceuticals! Bear in mind that the interests of pharmaceutical companies are very well served by having lifelong customers dependent upon their products.
- Hundreds of *billions* of dollars have been spent researching the 'cure' for cancer and the common cold and yet the solutions, it seems, remain as elusive as ever.
- Fundamentally, no headache was ever an aspirin deficiency, so how can a pharmaceutical hope to 'cure' the problem?
- Whilst the vaccination programme has taken credit for the decline in some diseases, this finding may actually be much more attributable to the introduction of proper sanitation and decent housing. Many also believe that the vaccination programme is at least partially responsible for many of our modern illnesses such as autism, ADHD, ADD, autoimmune diseases and asthma (see chapter 8).

The Trouble with Pharmaceutical Research and Development

Doctors give drugs of which they know little, into bodies, of which they know less, for disease of which they know nothing at all.

Voltaire

Pharmaceutical companies are ostensibly held to very high standards of testing before products are licensed and this is part of the problem. It now costs so much to trial and bring a drug to market that the pharmaceutical companies have to have unique rights for 20 years to recoup their investment. Natural products cannot be patented and so the search is always on to find a novel high-tech approach. The 'gold standard' of these drug trials is the double-blind trial where the participants do not know whether they are receiving the drug being investigated or a placebo and neither do the researchers. This is done to try and eliminate bias and the 'placebo effect'. This is the intriguing phenomenon whereby up to 70 per cent of the effect of a drug can be attributed to *what the patient expects that it will do for them* and patently is a very potent force.

Perhaps surprisingly, comparatively little research is ever undertaken into the interactions between the various over-the-counter and prescription medicines and yet it is not at all uncommon to find people taking cocktails of five or more drugs for a variety of ailments. Also, there is practically no research on the effects of pharmaceuticals in people with a variety of pre-existing conditions such as diabetes or asthma when the medication prescribed is for another illness. Finally, even a GlaxoSmithKline spokesman recently admitted that the vast majority of drugs only work in a *minority* of people.

Animal Testing

Another big issue in the research and testing of pharmaceuticals is the use of animals, most often rats or mice, as models for human physiology. The assumption is that our biochemistry is similar, but rats and mice are rodents, not apes like us, and just because a drug works in a rat does not mean it will work in humans and vice versa. After promising results in animals, the first drug trial in the UK in 2006 of TGN1412, manufactured by TeGenero, caused massive organ failure in the formerly healthy volunteers and left them fighting first for their lives and then to keep their extremities. Thalidomide too had appeared promising in animals only to have tragic and unforeseen consequences in humans. More recently, the arthritis drug Vioxx was withdrawn after causing up to 140,000 heart attacks and strokes in the USA. The US Food and Drug Administration (FDA) described it as 'the single greatest drug-safety catastrophe in the history of the world'. In fact, most experimental rats are male in whom the disease being studied is artificially induced and, in any event, these studies are only thought to predict adverse reactions in humans about 5 per cent of the time.

When it comes to pharmaceutical research there are the usual problems inherent in any study, but throw in considerations to do with funding, 'donations', regulatory bodies and the whole sticky mess of big business and, in this as in all things, 'Follow the money' is probably a good adage.

The Trouble with Medical Training

There is no question that there are some incredibly dedicated, good and bright people working both on the front line of medicine and behind the scenes, endeavouring to solve the world's health problems. However, there is a herd mentality which keeps unconventional thinkers in line and ensures agreement amongst the masses.

The problems, perhaps, begin with young medical students. They are bright, ambitious, hard-working and mostly young and fit, with little or no experience of being on the receiving end of the treatments they are likely to mete out, or indeed of the suffering involved in being ill. There is a massive amount of information to learn at medical school and there simply is no time for independent thought or questioning. They also trust and believe the authority figures who, in their turn, have been through the same process, and exams are essentially passed by parroting what they have learned. Many never stop to question the wisdom of the approach that they are taught, until it touches them or their family – usually decades later. Most medical students are also given practically no instruction about what is needed to maintain a body in health using nutrition. It would make no sense to a car mechanic to discount the possibility of the fuel being the cause of an engine malfunction – but this is what doctors do. And, as you probably appreciate, human bodies are infinitely and exquisitely more complex than the most sophisticated car.

Whilst it is true that you need to see it to believe it, it is also true that you need to believe it to be able to see it. The Native Americans were rumoured either not to have seen Columbus' ships as they approached or at least not to have understood what they were seeing because it was so far outside of their frame of reference. In the same way, the medical profession absolutely refuses to acknowledge the existence of some conditions for which the evidence is overwhelming, for example, overgrowth of the yeast Candida albicans, which many experts estimate to be at epidemic proportions in the developed world.

They also do not accept that some people cannot tolerate certain foods, which is counterintuitive to many. One consideration is that farming was introduced relatively recently in evolutionary terms (10,000 years ago) and with agriculture both dairy and grain products were introduced as staples of the diet. It appears that man may be fairly poorly equipped to digest these foodstuffs, both of which contain long-chain protein molecules, and these two foods are responsible for the lion's share of food intolerances. Another consideration is that man has adapted to his specific environment over long periods of time. Whilst an Inuit may be suited to a diet of blubber and fish, for example, a Bantu tribesman, used to eating corn (maize), meat and vegetables, might fare very badly on such a diet and vice versa.

Now that the body of medical knowledge has become so huge and complex, specialization means that everyone has a different piece of the puzzle and few now have a wider perspective. I know the whole time I was a dentist it never occurred to me to ask patients suffering with jaw joint problems whether they had digestive problems, for instance. I had my dental blinkers on (that had been carefully placed there by my dental schools) and I simply never considered the possibility that the cause was anything to do with – the body! I also both reassured patients about, and dismissed as being of no significance, sure signs of mercury toxicity such as a metallic taste and 'geographical tongue' (continent-like bald patches), because that was what I had been taught.

Medicine in the Real World

Doctors do not diagnose any more or look for causes. There isn't time. In the UK the consultation time is a few minutes per patient. I know in the whole time I consulted doctors about my failing health, not one examined me and indeed it was rare for any of them to actually even look at me (as opposed to their computer screen). As a result, doctors have come to depend very heavily on prescribing or requesting a laboratory test. This is because both procedures are quick and most people attending the doctor have come in the expectation of being given pills or being referred elsewhere. In fact, so keen are they to give out pharmaceutical drugs that they frequently prescribe antibiotics for infections they know to be viral. All members of the medical profession also need to be able to demonstrate that they have followed correct procedures and they place absolute faith in test results, which for a variety of reasons (examined in chapters 5 and 10) may be misplaced.

Doctors are also keen to prescribe relatively untried drugs preventatively, such as the widespread use of hormone replacement therapy (HRT). The chairman of the German Commission on the Safety of Medicines recently described HRT as 'the new thalidomide' and a recent paper in *The Lancet* (Lagro-Janssen et al., 2003) estimated that HRT had caused 20,000 cases of breast cancer in the past decade in the UK and many thousands of heart attacks and strokes. The profession also missed the fact that the prophylactic aspirin they were prescribing to prevent heart disease was causing more deaths from strokes than it was preventing from cardiovascular disease! Antibiotics, too, are proving to be far from the beneficial or benign drugs that they were once assumed to be. When administered during pregnancy they can cause profound birth defects; in childhood they can cause asthma and deafness and are responsible for 70,000 emergency admissions in the US every year.

All of the above relates to the proper practice of allopathic medicine, before we even touch on the thorny subject of unnecessary treatment and medical mistakes, which have affected nearly half the population respectively.

It is not that some people do not know what to do with the truth when
it is offered to them, but the tragic fate is to reach, after patient search, a
condition of mind-blindness in which the truth is not recognized, though
it stares you in the face.

Sir William Osler

What Allopathic Medicine Cannot Explain

The medical profession uses various words to legitimize (or disguise) the state of their
ignorance on some matters. Here are explanations of some medical terms that you may
or may not be familiar with:

- *Idiopathic*: This term is used to refer to a disease with a cause that modern
  medicine does not understand.
- *Chronic*: A disease that persists for a long time, will not usually spontaneously
  disappear and *cannot be cured* using allopathic modalities.
- *Iatrogenic*: This refers to a state of ill health or harmful consequences resulting
  from the actions of physicians or other health professionals and represents the
  leading cause of death in the US.
- *Psychosomatic*: This is an illness whose symptoms are believed to be caused by
  the mental processes of the sufferer and is usually applied where a physiological
  cause cannot be identified. Essentially, this term is used for illnesses that
  allopathic medicine doesn't understand and is a measure of our current
  ignorance. This term is often used to imply that the disease or symptom is
  imagined.
- *Incurable*: This word does not exist in any indigenous language and translates
  as 'I do not know how to cure you,' which is a wholly allopathic concept. The
  very word 'cancer' strikes fear into the hearts of many and being told by an
  expert in a white coat that you have a terminal illness may induce the *nocebo*
  effect. This is the flip side of the placebo effect whereby people get sicker and
  may even die because this is their deeply held expectation.
- *Spontaneous remission*: This refers to a sudden and dramatic improvement in a
  condition for reasons that modern medicine does not understand.

There are more things in heaven and earth, Horatio,
than are dreamt of in your philosophy.

Shakespeare

Chapter 3

The New Paradigm

You can't solve the problem with the same thinking
that created it.

Albert Einstein

If, then, the allopathic paradigm does not actually appear to be the answer to our woes and may, in fact, be contributing to the problems we face, where are the answers that we seek to be found? Well, the fact is that the answers are already here and many feel are being actively resisted by the established illness business. First, we need to examine the miracle of matter that is the human body.

Your Amazing Body

Most holistic therapists have a deep respect for the body and regard it as being amazing. The levels of organization and the sheer scale of the numbers involved are astounding. The first mind-boggling statistic is that the body is composed of *100 trillion intercommunicating cells.* Of these, ten million cells are replaced every second and each cell is believed to orchestrate over a hundred thousand biochemical reactions per second. The body generates three million nerve impulses and a million new nerve connections every second and there are over 100,000 km (60,000 miles) of lymphatic and blood vessels.

How does a fertilized egg ultimately organize itself into arms, heart, brain and ears and become a baby? How do molecules find and dock with their receptors? How do sperm 'know' which way to swim? We have approximately 26,000 genes and each one is believed to code for an enzyme, each of which may have hundreds of different shapes. However, it is estimated that less than 2 per cent of our genetic coding is active (some estimates are as low as 0.4 per cent). This means that we cannot account for the fantastic complexity of the body by physical means alone. Something that most holistic therapists agree on is that the body is not only utterly awe-inspiring, but that it is intelligent and animated by an unseen force.

A Bit of Quantum Physics

Most doctors probably have a Newtonian view of the universe, i.e. that the world consists of objects with distinct boundaries, where time progresses in an orderly and measured fashion. We now know that, although deceptively compelling, this model of reality is only partly true. There is another level of understanding where the visible universe is a manifestation of energy and information in the quantum domain. Einstein's famous equation $E = mc^2$ informs us that energy (E) equals mass (m) times the speed of light squared (c^2) – which is a very large and constant number. What this tells us is that matter (mass) is massively slowed down energy and the full implications of this discovery are only now starting to be realized. The small part of the universe that we currently understand is made of atoms and less than a trillionth of the atom consists of anything that could be described as matter. In fact, if the nucleus of the atom were the size of a peanut, the orbiting electron cloud would be the size of a football stadium. And if we were to collapse all the matter in the universe, it would fit inside a golf ball! As we investigate yet further, it seems possible that there is no such thing as matter at all, just the perception of matter by our senses. There is a further level of understanding some refer to as the 'field' and this is a domain of energy and information that is beyond time and space and from which everything emerges. It is the unseen organizing force behind all things and it is what binds quantum particles into atoms and animates and organizes our bodies. When someone dies the animating force leaves their body. However, the organs from this dead person can be taken and transplanted into another person's animating energy field – and live. How remarkable is that?

The Divine Matrix

It is now thought that not only is consciousness not the incidental and inexplicable result of millions of accidental evolutionary processes, but it is central to – and creating – our reality. Many eminent quantum physicists agree that we are involved in a very realistic holographic virtual reality simulation which is projected from hyperspace (higher dimensions). Further, your body hologram appears to be the result of your thought forms and to have been designed as the ultimate interactive learning environment! A hologram, by definition, contains the information for the whole in every piece just as every cell carries the genetic information for the whole. This is how reflexology, iridology and various other therapies work, because the pattern for the whole is contained in every part. In any event, you are not powerless, you are not an accident of evolution and you are not a victim of anything unless you choose to be. In fact, you are a divine being that is powerful beyond your wildest imaginings, and were you to truly believe it you could heal in an instant. However, we have been collectively conditioned over millennia to give our power away to external authorities, and to reclaim it requires conscious effort. We have given away control over our innate spirituality to organized religion, and control over our health to the medical profession. The placebo effect bears witness to the fact that we attribute our own healing power to the pills, but that it is our intention that heals.

The Holistic Model

> You never change things by fighting the existing reality. To change
> something, build a new model that makes the existing model obsolete.

Buckminster Fuller

The view of many holistic therapists is that, like a Russian doll, the physical body is the visible innermost body of several energy bodies that act as an energy template for the physical and 'step down' subtle universal energies into dense matter. Your body does not have an energy field around it – your body is *being created* by the energy field. The physical body is receiving instructions from this energy body, but until now, scientists have only been able to examine the physical half of the equation. Emotional and spiritual traumas are stored in these energy bodies and create energetic 'knots' in the energy field which are ultimately destined to appear in the physical body as disease. These may be long forgotten as far as your conscious mind is concerned, but have not been 'forgotten' by your cells or your energy bodies which exist outside of the concept of time.

The particular mechanism by which universal energies manifest in the physical involves the chakras, which are a series of seven main reducing transformers (often thought of as energy centres) running down the length of the spine. The chakras' function is to reduce extremely high vibrational energies to appear in what we have come to regard as the 'real', i.e. physical world as suggested by Einsteinian physics. They can be thought of as functioning a little like compact discs, storing information about emotional, mental and spiritual issues in addition to creating the physical body. The chakras can be seen by some sensitive people and their presence can be detected using various methods. These animating energies (referred to in China as 'chi' and in India as 'prana') are then routed along energy pathways known as meridians to all body organs and systems. Like an underground rail network, we can access these meridians where they surface although they also run deep within the body. The acupuncture points are where the physical and energetic bodies interface and have up to one-fifth the electrical resistance and several hundred times the electrical capacitance of the skin elsewhere and can be detected using electrical sensors. This mechanism explains why two individuals seemingly exposed to the same amounts of the same toxin may manifest different symptoms – one becoming infertile and another experiencing joint pain, for instance. Your physical body is always 'talking' to you and trying to illustrate the emotional, spiritual and mental issues that need resolving. Techniques such as homeopathy and vibrational remedies (such as Bach remedies) work in these energy bodies, which is why allopathic medicine is at a loss to understand how they can exert an effect.

So the good news is that by working on the spiritual, mental and emotional issues stored in your energy field, you can create the template for a healthy body. This requires that you do a lot of work on any issues that you think might be affecting your health. You may know what these issues are, but don't like to think about them and possibly can't imagine how they could be affecting you decades later. For some, the psyche perceived the causative issues as so traumatic that the memories have been completely buried and this presents a different problem. For you to get better, it is essential that you let go of everything that might be adversely affecting your health – all your grudges, resentments and grievances – and do it from the heart. Words are cheap and don't work.

> All truth passes through three stages: First, it is ridiculed; Second, it is
> violently opposed; and Third, it is accepted as self-evident.
>
> **Arthur Schopenhauer**

The Naturopathic Approach

Holistic medicine regards humans as not only biochemical beings, but also complex spiritual, emotional and mental beings, and it is hard to compare outcomes using the criteria employed by allopathic medicine. What the naturopathic and holistic world is saying is that the causes of illness are different in every person, although there may be common themes. One person may have heart disease because of some early trauma such as having a parent die. Another may have the identical condition because they have a genetic enzyme deficiency. In yet another it may be a deficiency of, or a high individual requirement for, a particular mineral. Since the causes are different in each case, the treatment appropriate to each individual must be different too – and tailored to fit.

> **It's supposed to be a secret, but I'll tell you anyway. We doctors do nothing. We only help and encourage the doctor within.**
>
> **Dr Albert Schweitzer**

Your body is self-healing. You break a leg and (provided it is set properly) it will heal. You cut yourself and the skin regrows. You get an infection and you run a fever, which both kills the invading organisms and turbo-charges your body's immune response. Encouragingly, 98 per cent of your body will be replaced in the next six months. However, when someone does not heal and progresses to disease, the naturopathic model likens this to an iceberg where the symptoms are the visible part of the iceberg – and the part that allopathic medicine has studied and named. However, beneath the surface lies the nine-tenths of the iceberg that is a body toxic with chemicals and microbes and compromised by structural issues – and underlying all these factors are past emotional traumas. As you address these causes of your symptoms and resolve these issues one by one, the iceberg gets smaller and the symptoms – the 'disease' – melt away.

Supplements and Herbs

The pharmaceutical companies are, possibly understandably, irked by what they see as less rigorous standards of licensing for food supplements and herbal medicines. However, there are a couple of major differences. One is that many of these herbs have effectively had a 'clinical trial' (albeit uncontrolled) lasting hundreds, if not thousands of years, and their actions and cautions are well understood. The second conceptual difference is that the allopathic medical world is very attached to the idea of the 'magic bullet' – identifying one active ingredient with pharmacological effect. Many herbs contain hundreds of ingredients and it is the synthesis of these that creates the therapeutic effect. It is like watching a winning football team and being forced to pick one winning player. Many pharmaceuticals have been derived from, or are patentable copies of herbs anyway – possibly even the majority.

Goals of Treatment

The goal of treatment has to be to aid the body in detoxifying, whilst assisting the body's efforts to rebuild using means as natural as possible, i.e. the naturopathic approach. Bear in mind that it has probably taken you many years to get from health to reading this book. As a consequence, you need to expect that it will take you at least six months of effort to start making inroads into your condition. In fact, it probably takes at least a year of determined detoxification for every decade of original 'toxification', so a long-term commitment is required. The improvements gained, however, are lasting. There is no truer adage than 'If you keep on doing what you've been doing, you'll keep on getting what you've been getting.' Your body is begging you to do things differently. The good news is that you can address the fundamental causes of your ill health. The bad news is that whilst fairly simple, none of this is easy. An absolutely unshakable commitment to getting well and doing everything necessary is going to be required. This may include changing lifetime patterns of behaviour and will certainly involve eating good nutritious food, exercising and drinking lots of water. The fact is that *health is primitive* and is not a function of high-tech wizardry or complex synthetic chemicals. There is an enormous difference between relying on daily medication to cope and actually enjoying feelings of well-being and enthusiasm about your life and what each day can bring. You may have become so used to managing your illness that you may not even realize what a big prize true health and well-being really are. Keep them in sight at all times and particularly when you may be flagging on the road to recovery.

Chapter 4
The Basics

Fatigue-related syndromes are complicated conditions that confound quite a lot of the doctors and others who have made a detailed study of them. In order to recover, you are going to need to understand the basics of how the body functions in health, what has gone wrong and why, and what you need to do to heal. This chapter covers the basics on how the various body systems should work and in chapter 7 we examine how these systems are affected in FRS. If science passed you by at school, well, here is a whistle-stop tour and if you are a therapist or have already read widely around this subject and are confident that you have a good grasp of basic physiology, feel free to skip or scan this section.

The Building Blocks of Life
Atoms

Everything in the known universe is made of atoms which are spheres of energy that are 99.9999 per cent space. They have a nucleus in the centre that contains particles that are neutral, but have some weight (neutrons), and particles that have no weight but carry positive charge (protons). Around this dense 'core' are little packets of negatively charged electrons held in their orbits by the pull of the nucleus. These electrons prefer to orbit as opposing pairs and atoms are most stable when the outermost shell is full of electrons. There are 92 naturally occurring elements and what gives any element its identity is the unique number of protons and neutrons in the nucleus. Thirty-four of these elements are essential for life with another third being 'conditionally' essential and the remaining third proving toxic. The periodic table lists the elements by increasing atomic weight and attempts to group elements that have similar properties, mostly because they have the same number of electrons in their outer shell.

The Cell

The basic building block of the body is the cell and to understand some of what occurs in disease, you need to understand a little of how the cell operates in health. The same genetic material is held in the nucleus of most of the body's cells. Different parts of this are activated in different tissues such as the brain and the liver, which makes those cells unique. The cell is surrounded by a cell membrane which is largely made of fats and this makes the cells waterproof to some extent. The membrane has receptors embedded in it that are specific for certain hormones, neurotransmitters or other compounds and these act as the 'doors' into the cell. When substances dock with their particular receptors, a process is set in motion within the cell, or a specific substance is permitted entry into the cell. The cell contains various organelles (little organs) suspended in watery gel called cytosol that all have different functions, and all these organelles (including the nucleus) have membranes that contain receptors too. All cells are suspended in a salt-water environment from which they obtain their nutrients and spew their waste products and it is this that interfaces with the circulatory system. Lysosomes are a specific kind of cell organelle that contain digestive enzymes that are used to destroy defunct organelles or even the whole cell and have been termed 'suicide bags'. The compounds that specific cells synthesize are also released into the intercellular matrix after little sacs migrate to the cell membrane and fuse with it. In the case of the thyroid gland this substance would be thyroxine (a thyroid hormone) and in the case of the pancreas it could be pancreatic enzyme. Recent research has determined that much of the intelligence of the cell and organelles relates to the activities of their respective membranes and not to the genetic code as previously assumed.

The Genetic Code

The genetic material is held primarily in the nucleus in the form of deoxyribonucleic acid (DNA), which is a long and elegant molecule structured like a coiled ladder. Each cell contains 2m (6ft) of DNA and the total amount in every human would go around the world five million times! The upright backbone of the molecule supports the 'rungs' which are composed of two complementary sugars and it is just four of these sugars that code for all of the information required to make a human. The DNA ladder can temporarily 'unzip', allowing counterpart sugars to dock onto the exposed 'rungs'. Then this small portion of the genetic code is transported in the form of messenger RNA (mRNA) which shuttles to small organelles known as ribosomes where this code is 'read' and a particular protein assembled. If one side of the DNA ladder is broken, then the damage can be repaired using the remaining strand as a template. However, if both strands are broken this damage cannot be repaired and this may lead to cancer or a birth defect depending upon the tissue affected.

Energy Production

The main energy source within the body is a compound called adenosine tri-phosphate (ATP) and this is synthesized within the cell, mostly from the carbohydrates that we eat. This process occurs inside an organelle known as a mitochondrion, of which there are a thousand on average in each cell. The mitochondria synthesize ATP from glucose and oxygen and generate waste carbon dioxide in the process. The ATP is then exported from the mitochondrion to another location within the cell where its extra phosphate bond is broken to produce adenosine di-phosphate (ADP) with the release of energy, which can be used by the cell. The spent ADP then returns to the mitochondrion for recycling back into ATP and so the process goes on. The average person makes almost their body weight in ATP every day and for this reason, the mitochondria and their health are of vital importance in energy production. Perhaps critically, the mitochondria are also about twenty times more sensitive to toxicity than other cell organelles.

Free Radicals

Our growing understanding of free radical damage is probably one of the greatest recent breakthroughs. Free radicals are unstable and greedy atoms or molecules with an unpaired electron in their outer shell. The free radical is disposed to steal an electron from another molecule, which in turn snatches an electron from another molecule, and this process can start a whole cascade of devastation. The more recent term reactive oxygen species (ROS) is now more properly used because not all damaging oxygen species are free radicals. An antioxidant is a generous and stable molecule that can donate an electron to the hungry ROS and not be adversely affected itself.

The generation of energy using the oxygen that we breathe inevitably produces ROS within the cell – like sparks from a flame. Other factors such as poor nutrition, drug use, smoking and sunbathing also generate ROS. The damage created is constantly being mopped up, provided that the ROS produced are within reasonable limits and that the person has consumed adequate quantities of antioxidants in their diet. Problems arise when the diet is deficient and/or the system is overloaded with ROS, in which case permanent damage starts to occur to the cells that cannot be repaired. The mitochondria are furnaces of energy production and any damage sustained by the mitochondria will lead to compromised function – which means compromised energy production. ROS damage is thought to lead to ageing and degenerative illnesses and may cause cancer or birth defects if the genetic material is affected.

Understanding the Body

The following is a brief description of the various body systems. It should be understood, however, that these distinctions are a purely artificial construction to aid understanding, and that in reality every cell in the body is communicating with, and is dependent upon, every other cell. It is just not possible that one part can become diseased whilst the rest of the body remains healthy as per the dictates of allopathic medicine. On the contrary, *the whole system becomes compromised* and whilst it has a remarkable capacity to compensate for adversely affected organs or systems, this is not infinite and eventually one of these will fail first.

The Digestive System

Essentially, we humans are just elaborate and mobile feeding tubes! Unlike single cell creatures that can absorb nutrients from, and expel waste products into, their surroundings, we are large and complex. For this reason we are designed to take in a supply of food at one end of a tube, absorb the nutrients from it and then excrete the waste through the other end. This tube is variously referred to as the gut, intestine, gastrointestinal tract or alimentary canal and is technically an external surface. Of course, there's a little more to it than that – so here's a simplified version of what your intestines do for you.

The Intestines

As we chew food, we mince it up with our teeth and coat it with the first of many digestive enzymes which are present in saliva. This mixture, known as a bolus, is then swallowed and passes down to the stomach where it spends some hours being churned and bathed in more digestive enzymes. The stomach contents at this point are very acidic and this helps to break down proteins, to kill any swallowed organisms and to activate the protein-digesting enzyme, pepsin. Protein-digesting enzymes are produced in an inactive form and then activated *in situ*, otherwise they would digest the very organs that contain or produce them. When it is ready, this semi-liquid purée known as chyme is discharged into the small intestine. Here it meets almost immediately and simultaneously with bile from the gall bladder and other digestive enzymes from the pancreas. Between them these secretions essentially complete the chemical breakdown of the food into nutrients that can then be utilized by the body.

Your small intestine is over 7m long (23ft) and is coiled and folded in the central part of your abdomen, behind your navel. The chyme is moved along by a wave-like squeezing contraction of the muscular walls known as peristalsis. The small intestine lining has finger-like projections known as villi which are covered in further velvety projections known as microvilli and this means that the surface area of the intestine is absolutely enormous, with one square centimetre representing an area the size of a tennis court. The majority of the nutrients are absorbed directly into either the bloodstream or the lymphatic system through this vast internal membrane. These nutrients are then transported to the liver and on to the rest of the body to be used as fuel and building materials. The majority of the bile is reabsorbed in the terminal part of the small intestine and recycled back to the liver in the portal vein and this is known as the enterohepatic circulation ('entero' refers to the intestine and 'hepatic' to liver) or bile loop.

The chyme then moves from the small intestine into the large intestine (or colon) – so called because of their respective girths. The large intestine is 1.6m long (5ft) and passes up the right-hand side of the body, across the abdomen (above the navel) and down the left-hand side of the torso to the rectum and anus. Where the small intestine empties into the large intestine, there is a valve known as the ileocaecal valve (pronounced il-ee-o-see-kal). This valve regulates the passage of chyme into the large intestine and also prevents the backflow of contaminated bowel contents into the small intestine where they would be absorbed. This valve is located halfway between the right hip crest and the navel and when dysfunctional can often be painful – a pain that can often unfortunately be mistaken for appendicitis.

The large intestine is inhabited by several kilos of 500 different species of bacteria – which is ten times as many bacteria as there are cells in the body! These friendly bacteria complete the digestion of the remaining food, produce vitamins and minerals that are absorbed and used by the body and are responsible for 25 per cent of detoxification. The colon is also thought to house 75 per cent of the immune system since it is the biggest area of exposure to the environment. Once in the colon, water is absorbed from the chyme to form a solid mass of waste, which is packaged, ready for defecation. Mucous helps to lubricate the waste and protect the body from the toxic stool.

The Liver

The liver constantly filters the blood and has at least 500 and possibly thousands of different functions. The liver detoxifies; redirects nutrients to other parts of the body; synthesizes bile; removes ageing blood cells and any parasites from circulation and generally monitors blood contents. Your liver is critical to your overall health and its function is usually severely compromised in all chronic diseases. Fortunately, the liver has a remarkable capacity for regeneration and given the right nutrients it is possible to nurse your liver back to health.

The liver processes toxins through two different biochemical phases. The first of these (phase I) is known as hydroxylation and this is where substances are made water-soluble and often results in temporarily making a toxic substance even more toxic. The second phase (phase II) is known as conjugation, whereby the liver adds various substances to the products of phase I. There are six different biochemical pathways in this second phase. These processes have a high requirement for minerals, vitamins and nutrients which, if deficient, mean that the body is unable to adequately detoxify. 'Pathological detoxifiers' are people who can adequately process substances through phase I liver detoxification but are then unable to process a substance through phase II for lack of an enzyme or mineral, for instance.

The Gall Bladder
The gall bladder acts as a storage organ which concentrates the bile that the liver is constantly producing. The gall bladder contracts (when chemically signalled to do so) just as the chyme leaves the stomach and enters the small intestine. The function of bile is to emulsify fats (make them into little droplets), so that other enzymes can work to digest them. It is also the body's favoured method of excreting any toxic fat-soluble substances and large particles, such as parasites.

The Pancreas
The pancreas is a dual-purpose organ in the upper left of the abdomen. It produces digestive enzymes which empty into the small intestine along with bile from the gall bladder. These pancreatic enzymes help to break down proteins and complete digestion of all foodstuffs. The other role of the pancreas is as an endocrine organ and this is addressed below.

The Endocrine System
The prefix 'endo-' means 'within' and here it refers to a system of widely separated inter-communicating and interdependent glands within the body that release hormones directly into the circulation. These circulating hormones act as messengers that find their way to a specific target tissue receptor and cause some sort of effect. The whole endocrine system is very finely balanced and the glands compensate for each other. This means that one dysfunctional gland can ultimately affect the entire endocrine system.

The endocrine system consists of the following organs:

- the testes in men and the ovaries in women, which produce sex hormones;
- the thyroid gland, which controls metabolism and growth;
- the parathyroid glands, which regulate mineral balance;
- the thymus, which plays a key role in the immune response;
- the pancreas, which regulates blood sugar;

- the adrenal glands, which are primarily responsible for the stress response but also have other functions.

Orchestrating all this activity are three controlling glands in the brain: the pineal, the hypothalamus and the pituitary gland.

All of these glands are affected to a greater or lesser extent in FRS, however the thyroid and adrenal glands are invariably involved along with the hypothalamus in the brain and for this reason we will examine them in a little more detail.

The Thyroid Gland

The thyroid gland is a small gland at the front and base of the throat. It mainly produces inactive thyroxine (sometimes known as T4), which is then converted into its active form of tri-iodothyronine (T3) in the tissues and liver. Thyroid hormones are a kind of growth hormone and govern the metabolism in practically all the body's tissues and also enhance the effects of other hormones.

The Adrenal Glands

The adrenal glands are small glands that sit on top of the kidneys and are located under the ribs in the back. They have several different and important functions, but are primarily responsible for our response to stress. The adrenal glands produce (amongst many other hormones) adrenaline (epinephrine), which provides an immediate and short-term response to stress and the steroid hormone, cortisol, which provides a medium-to-long-term stress response.

Both the adrenal and thyroid glands receive their instructions from hormones released by the pituitary gland in the brain under the direction of the hypothalamus, which contains sensors that are constantly monitoring all hormone levels. These are respectively known as the hypothalamus-pituitary-adrenal axis (HPA axis) and the hypothalamus-pituitary-thyroid axis (HPT axis) and it may be the master glands, these axes and/or the whole endocrine system that are compromised in FRS and not just one component.

The Hypothalamus

The hypothalamus is a highly organized collection of nerve tissue at the base of the brain that is about the size of an almond. The small size belies the overarching importance of this gland which processes information gathered from the five senses and various regions of the central nervous system. It also constantly monitors levels of hormones and other substances in the circulation and the cerebrospinal fluid (the fluid that surrounds the brain and spinal cord). The hypothalamus then relays information to the adjacent pituitary gland which releases hormones into the circulation. It also controls the autonomic nervous system which is the 'automatic' nervous system that controls all functions that operate beneath conscious awareness. In these various capacities, the hypothalamus acts as the interface between the mind and body and indirectly controls virtually every cell. In this way variables such as temperature and blood pressure are maintained within narrow parameters by means of constant adjustments that result in the seemingly steady state of homeostasis.

It is hard to overemphasize the importance of the hypothalamus in maintaining health since it controls such functions as sleep/wake cycles; the immune response; body temperature; hunger and appetite; urination and defecation, and testicular and ovarian function. Were that not enough, the hypothalamus also governs emotional behaviour including feelings of anger or rage, sexual behaviour and feelings of either pleasure and energy or emptiness and depression. It also plays a key role in enhancing memory and learning and, perhaps significantly, has a different structure in men and women and also differs between heterosexual and homosexual individuals. The protective blood–brain barrier is perforated adjacent to the hypothalamus to allow for monitoring of blood contents and excretion of substances directly into the circulation. As a consequence, the hypothalamus is the most vulnerable part of the brain to toxic insult.

The Nervous System

For convenience, the nervous system is regarded as being composed of the central and peripheral nervous systems. The central nervous system includes the brain and spinal cord, and the peripheral nervous system is the system of nerves that connect it to distant body parts. These peripheral nerves can be either sensory or motor nerves. Sensory nerves convey information to the central nervous system concerning the outside world (via the special senses such as sight and hearing) and from within the body (such as pain or joint positions). Motor nerves relay instructions from the central nervous system to the tissues and usually cause the body to respond in some way to the information it has received from the sensory system. Whilst these signals pass along the length of the nerve using electrical means they ultimately stimulate the release of chemicals known as neurotransmitters at their terminal end. There are over a hundred of these different chemicals which either transmit the signal to another nerve at a 'junction' or produce some other sort of effect.

The Brain

The brain is quite literally the 'nerve centre' of the body and whilst it accounts for 2 per cent of our body weight, it receives 20 per cent of our circulating blood and oxygen delivered by approximately tens of thousands of miles/kilometres of blood vessels. It constantly processes the millions of incoming pieces of information to keep all the body parameters operating within narrow limits. Your brain consists of about 100 billion nerve cells (neurones), each of which has between 1,000 to 10,000 synapses (connections). The living brain has the consistency of blancmange in that it is 85 per cent water and of the remainder, two-thirds is fat. Neurones have more mitochondria and a greater demand for both glucose and oxygen weight-for-weight than any other tissue. The brain is protected from the circulation by the blood–brain barrier which is composed of membranes and their associated cells and is also suspended in a watery fluid known as cerebrospinal fluid. This fluid supplies essential nutrients and provides an additional layer of protection from the chemicals, microbes and/or parasites that may be present in the blood. The body will always prioritize the function of its two most vital organs – the heart and brain – at the expense of other less 'essential' organs or tissues such as the joints or the uterus.

Regions of the Brain

The central nervous system is arranged in three layers. The 'reptilian' brain responsible for survival responses is innermost, enclosed by the limbic system or emotional brain. Outermost is the conscious or thinking brain. The limbic system incorporates several structures at the base of the brain including the amygdala (a small cluster of nerve cell nuclei), the hypothalamus and the hippocampus, and these intercommunicate with the sense of smell in the reptilian brain. The hippocampus plays an important role in short-term memory and orientation in space and is one of the first regions to be affected in Alzheimer's disease. The amygdala is involved in emotional responses and memory; the information processed here is not filtered by the conscious mind. The history of all unpleasant events is thought to be recorded in the left amygdala; all projected events (including nightmares) are thought to originate in the right amygdala. The amygdala is involved in activating the hypothalamus and therefore indirectly in the stimulation of the autonomic nervous system (see below) and the production of stress hormones. The reticular activating system (RAS) is a region where the spinal cord and brain meet which contains 70 per cent of the brain's nerve cells, and it has come under particular scrutiny in relation to FRS. It acts as a filter between conscious and unconscious awareness and is associated with motivation, arousal, sleep-wake cycles, muscle tone, heart rate, breathing and modulating pain.

The Autonomic Nervous System

The autonomic nervous system (ANS) monitors and controls all the automatic functions necessary for life that occur beneath conscious awareness. Eighty per cent of the ANS is thought to be devoted to sensory, incoming information and 20 per cent to regulating processes like digestion, maintenance of blood pressure, breathing, urination, sweating and penile erection. The autonomic nervous system is governed by the emotional right brain and is composed of two opposing systems, the parasympathetic (PSNS) and sympathetic nervous systems (SNS). These work respectively like the brakes (PSNS) and the accelerator/gas (SNS) in a car. There are so many branches of the ANS involved in digestion that this network is often referred to as the 'second brain'. This system is also responsible for sexual sensation, sexual arousal and erection of the penis in the male and engorgement of the vagina and clitoris in the female. Adrenaline (epinephrine) produced by the adrenal glands also potentiates the actions of the sympathetic nervous system.

The Lymphatic and Immune Systems

The lymphatic and immune systems are closely connected and are often regarded as different components of the same system.

The Lymphatic System

As you probably already appreciate, the blood is pumped by the heart inside a closed system of vessels known as the circulatory system. This system delivers oxygen (from your lungs) and nutrients (from the intestines) to your tissues, and then transports away waste products. These waste products are then either filtered by the liver and eliminated in the bile or excreted by the kidneys as urine. The waste gases such as carbon dioxide are eliminated by the lungs. What you may not appreciate is that the circulatory system is intimately connected to a parallel and larger system of lymphatic vessels which accompany the blood vessels one way only from the tissues. These lymphatic vessels both drain away excess fluid and also filter the lymph produced through a series of lymph nodes, ultimately to return the lymph back into the circulation in the chest. The lymph nodes monitor the lymph and activate an appropriate immune response if anything untoward is detected. Unlike the circulatory system, the lymphatic system has no central pump. Instead it relies upon the pulsing of the walls of the larger vessels, the movement of adjacent muscles and arteries and a series of internal valves that prevent backflow. There are also several clusters of lymphatic tissue that are open to the surface of the body in various locations and these include the tonsils and lymphatic patches in the intestines known as Peyer's patches.

The Immune System

This is an immensely elegant, complex and sophisticated system of initiating and terminating responses to perceived threats, which can include bacteria or foreign proteins from a substance such as an egg – in which case the response would be regarded as an allergy. It comprises the white blood cells (leukocytes) which have been broadly grouped into those that have many lysosomes (which appear granular when dyed) and those that do not. The granular leukocytes include neutrophils (which engulf and digest microbes and debris), eosinophils (which attack parasites and are involved in allergy) and basophils (which are also involved in allergy and release histamine). The non-granular leukocytes are known as lymphocytes and originate in the bone marrow, forming two main groups which are then activated either in the thymus gland, for which reason they are known as T-lymphocytes, or in the bone and classified as B-lymphocytes. These two arms of the lymphocyte system of cells then interact to aid one another in both initiating and terminating immune responses and in defending the body against microbes, fungi and rogue cancer cells. They also act to keep a 'library' of previously encountered proteins for future reference. A third group of lymphocytes are referred to as natural killer cells and these combat viruses and cancerous cells. The entire system works on the basis of being able to identify cells marked as 'self' from those that are 'non-self'.

The newborn baby's immune system is primed by the first milk that the mother produces (known as colostrum) and thereafter by breast milk until the young infant's system can be independent. The organ believed by many holistic therapists to orchestrate the immune response is the thymus gland which lies behind the breastbone. Allopathic medicine, however, regards this organ as not serving any important function after acting as a stopgap in the newborn until they can get their own immune system up and running.

The immune system is invariably compromised in fatigue-related syndromes. An underactive immune system will not be able to mount an effective response to infections, which can then become recurrent or chronic. The creation of a cancerous cell is not a rare occurrence at all. In fact, at any moment we all probably have dozens, if not hundreds, of cancerous cells in our bodies. An efficient immune system, however, will detect and destroy these cells whereas an underactive immune system may either not recognize these rogue cells or be unable to destroy them. It is for this reason that many consider cancer to be a consequence of an underactive immune system. Equally, an overactive immune system may attack seemingly innocent cells flagged as 'self' as in so-called 'autoimmune' diseases.

Detoxification

Channels of Excretion

If your body wishes to excrete a toxic substance it has the relatively few options outlined below at its disposal.

Intestines

Most fat-soluble wastes, toxic metals and other fragments such as parasite, fungal or bacterial remains are extracted from the circulating blood by the liver and ultimately excreted as bile in the faeces. This toxic bile may be reabsorbed if there is insufficient fibre or poor peristalsis, resulting in further concentration of toxins in the bile and compromising gall bladder function. Flatulence is the expelling of toxic gases produced by bacterial or fungal fermentation along with swallowed gases and this may be used as a route of excretion of toxic gas wastes.

Kidneys

Water-soluble wastes are excreted as urine by the kidneys which filter 180 litres (320 pints) of fluid out of the blood every day. The body then selectively draws back 99 per cent of the resulting fluid under hormonal instructions as to what it needs to retain. Due to the volumes of fluid processed, any water-soluble toxins in circulation such as toxic metals will rapidly have an adverse effect on the kidneys. The resulting urine is temporarily stored in the bladder until it is convenient to urinate.

Skin and Mucosa

Some toxins are excreted through the skin as sweat. This route means that the toxins are unlikely to be reabsorbed as can happen with elimination via both the kidneys and intestine. This may also be the preferred route if the other excretion routes are blocked, or possibly if the toxins are stored more superficially in body fat. Substances can also be secreted through the mucosal lining of the vagina, mouth and nose. Tears may be a minor route of excretion.

Lungs

Vapours and gases may be excreted via the lungs and this may occasionally produce foul-smelling breath.

Men Only

Seminal fluid may be used as a minor route of excretion.

Women Only

In women, the body also uses the uterus for storage and excretion of toxins in the monthly blood flow. Unfortunately, this propensity also means that pregnant mothers are estimated to pass two-thirds of their body burden of toxins into their developing foetus.

Toxin Storage

If these detoxification routes are blocked, then the body resorts to temporarily storing toxins in body cavities such as the joints, sinuses and muscles until such time as nutrients are available to excrete the toxins. Body fat is also a convenient toxin storage depot and as such may prove extremely resistant to removal using all the usual means. The body will always try to protect the vital organs and so another favoured technique is to store toxins in the extremities and then restrict the blood supply to those regions and this can lead to cold hands and feet, fungal finger- and toenails and Reynaud's-type symptoms. A naturopathic principle is that the body attempts to excrete or store toxins superficially, at first resulting in symptoms such as eczema. Then, over time the toxins are stored in deeper and deeper body compartments so that symptoms progress from asthma and/or hyperactivity to migraines, for instance. With time, irritable bowel syndrome may transition into tiredness and ultimately to end-stage debilitating illnesses such as multiple sclerosis or rheumatoid arthritis. Many think that they 'grew out of' asthma or eczema, but in reality the problem has just gone deeper to manifest at a later date as another more chronic disease. Conversely, as toxins are brought out of deep storage, they may be excreted superficially through the skin.

Chapter 5
Defining Fatigue-Related Syndromes

Disease is the warning, and therefore the friend – not the enemy – of mankind.

Dr George S Weger

Chronic Fatigue Syndrome

Fatigue is an extremely common symptom, with one in five of the population and up to three-quarters of patients attending their physician complaining of persistent fatigue. However, when using the term CFS, 'chronic' means that the condition has gone on for some time, 'fatigue' refers to a debilitating and profound fatigue and 'syndrome' to a specific pattern of symptoms and signs. Broadly, a sign is something a doctor could observe and a symptom is something the sufferer is likely to report, such as insomnia.

Chronic fatigue syndrome (CFS) is the current term used for the disorder formerly known as myalgic encephalomyelitis (ME) since 1956. The term myalgic encephalomyelitis was coined after people who had contracted viral infections were demonstrated to have what was thought to be residual inflammation of the brain accompanied by changes in the spinal cord fluid. As such, ME has been recognized by the World Health Organization as a disease of the central nervous system since 1969. This name has now fallen out of favour because it is thought to be both inaccurate and misleading. This disorder has also been referred to derogatively as 'Yuppie flu' and more recently suggested terms include chronic fatigue immune dysfunction syndrome (CFIDS) and neuro-endocrine-immune dysfunction syndrome (NDS).

The primary presenting symptom of CFS is fatigue and according to the 1994 Center for Disease Control criteria (http://www.cdc.gov/cfs) it can only be diagnosed after six months of experiencing new and incapacitating fatigue that cannot be attributed to another medical cause. The fatigue should also not be improved by rest and should be accompanied by at least four of the following:

- Impairment of short-term memory and concentration
- A sore throat
- Tender lymph nodes
- Muscle pain
- Multi-joint pain
- Headaches of a new type, pattern or severity
- Unrefreshing sleep or insomnia
- Fatigue lasting more than 24 hours after exertion

There are a host of other associated signs and symptoms which many CFS sufferers experience and these will be examined in more detail in chapter 7. The condition is not new, with descriptions of similar disorders dating back to antiquity and certainly being recognized in recent centuries.

Fibromyalgia Syndrome

Fibromyalgia or fibromyalgia syndrome (FM or FMS) is a chronic syndrome which is also characterized by chronic fatigue and many of the other symptoms of CFS. In fact, 70 per cent of all fibromyalgia sufferers experience overwhelming fatigue and 95 per cent meet the diagnostic criteria for CFS. However, in fibromyalgia the primary presenting symptom is muscle, joint and/or bone pain which often occurs in the shoulder, back and/or neck regions. To get an official diagnosis of fibromyalgia the sufferer must have experienced widespread pain (in more than one quadrant – where the body is divided into four 'quarters' above and below the waist, right and left) for at least three months. In 1990 the American College of Rheumatology developed criteria for the diagnosis of fibromyalgia including the presence of tenderness or pain in 11 or more of 18 specific points on the body. It is valuable to note that these definitions and those listed above for diagnosis of CFS are the official medical research criteria and are not intended for clinical application. Within the population at large, up to one in eight people complain of chronic widespread pain that does not meet the strict criteria for fibromyalgia.

Fibromyalgia affects nine times as many females as males, occurs in up to 6 per cent of the general population and is twice as common as rheumatoid arthritis. It is most commonly diagnosed between the ages of 20 and 50 years old and reaches a peak between 55 and 60 years of age, although it can start in childhood. Again, while terminologies may change, the condition was recognized in the 1800s as muscular rheumatism and renamed fibrositis in 1904 with many other terms suggested since.

Multiple Chemical Sensitivity

Many sufferers of multiple chemical sensitivity (MCS) also have a chronic condition bearing many of the hallmarks of CFS or fibromyalgia. However, their primary presenting problem is an oversensitive or deranged immune system that responds to many unrelated and environmental chemicals.

I have spared you many of the complex terminologies here which all serve to demonstrate how confused the medical profession is about this issue. Just like the blind men who felt the elephant and all formed a completely different picture of the beast, these conditions are all, in fact, manifestations of the same or similar problem(s). It is for this reason I refer to these conditions collectively as fatigue-related syndromes (FRS) throughout this book.

The Scale of the Problem

Sadly, if you are suffering with CFS you are not alone. It is estimated that at least 300,000 people in the UK and up to two million people in the USA have been diagnosed with CFS and the real figure of those suffering is probably much higher. One estimate puts the total number of people affected worldwide by chronic fatigue syndrome alone at over 90 million. Since only one in five people with CFS are believed to get a diagnosis, this potentially places the total number of people affected by CFS at around the half billion mark worldwide. There are also tens of millions of people with other, similar, fatiguing illnesses who do not fully meet the strict criteria for a diagnosis of CFS. Nearly a quarter of patients attending their doctors, for instance, complain of persistent tiredness or feeling 'tired all the time' (TATT).

The diagnosis of CFS embraces a wide range of disabilities from a mild persistent fatigue with post-exertion symptoms through to sufferers being completely bedridden and unable to care for themselves. Many have a compromised ability to function, an inability to perform strenuous duties and the need to carefully pace themselves with frequent rest periods. The typical pattern may also be patchy and unpredictable with sufferers having 'good' days where they are able to function quite well, followed typi-cally by 'bad' days where they may need to take to their beds.

The levels of debility seen in some individuals affected by CFS are recognized as being comparable to those experienced in conditions such as multiple sclerosis, rheumatoid arthritis and even terminal cancer. As a consequence, many sufferers are unable to participate in what others would consider 'normal' activities and may experience profound social isolation. Sadly, the most infirm also often receive the least support from health and social services, possibly because they simply become too sick to fight the system or to demand the help that they need. One study found that CFS patients received worse social support than disease-free cancer patients or healthy patients!

For most sufferers there will be no *spontaneous* recovery. Approximately half of sufferers may experience some improvement over time; equally one in five sufferers' condition will deteriorate further. If you have experienced chronic fatigue for more than six months, the medical profession gives you less than a 2 per cent chance of recovery. Some people become able to work, for instance, but are never truly well.

Tests

At this time, there are no accepted tests for chronic fatigue syndrome. The diagnosis is made on the basis of signs, symptoms, examination and eliminating other potential causes of the patient's symptoms. The doctor should take a detailed history, consider the possibility that symptoms are a side effect of current medication and then perform a thorough physical and mental examination. Well, that's the textbook version anyway. They should then order a battery of laboratory screening tests to exclude the following potential causes before an official diagnosis of CFS is made:

- Endocrine disorders such as hypothyroidism (underactive thyroid); Addison's disease (underactive adrenal glands); Cushing's disease (overactive adrenal glands) or diabetes
- Sub-acute or chronic infections such as Lyme disease or mononucleosis
- Deficiencies such as vitamin B12 deficiency; ferritin, iron, folic acid and/or calcium deficiencies and various anaemias
- Digestive disorders such as coeliac disease, gluten intolerance, ulcers and/or tumours of the intestines
- Diseases or infections of the heart, liver or kidneys
- Temperomandibular (jaw) joint disorder (TMJ or TMD)
- Polycystic ovary syndrome (PCOS)
- Various autoimmune conditions such as rheumatological or muscle disorders
- Central nervous system disorders and multiple sclerosis
- Psychiatric conditions such as major depressive or eating disorders
- Alcohol or substance abuse

- Finally, a ragbag of cancers; metabolic syndromes; immune system dysfunction; primary sleep disorders and severe obesity

Well, as you can see that is quite a list, and most patients and most doctors do not exclude all of the above. You should, however, go and see your doctor to rule out the possibility of your symptoms being due to one of these causes, although even if this is the case, the information in the following chapters will help you too. You can throw an awful lot of money at having test after test done in the hope of receiving an accurate diagnosis. All this tends to do is leave you possibly poorer, older, probably sicker and even more desperate – with a fat file of test results that all demonstrate that there is nothing wrong with you. Unfortunately, this adds nothing to your under-standing and tends to add to the belief of the medical profession that the illness is psychosomatic and that you are neurotic. No test is definitive, but some tests may prove more instructive than others, including fractionated urinary porphyrin or toxic metal analysis, and blood tests that demonstrate the presence of various viruses, yeasts, toxic metals or endocrine dysfunction. Provocation tests such as the Kelmer test involve taking various chelating agents (chemicals that pull heavy metals from storage for excretion) and then monitoring urine samples; these may indicate specific toxicity and be acceptable to some insurers. Some practitioners also find various mitochondrial function and immune profiles useful. Ultimately, however, the only tests of any value would be to have either a brain or kidney biopsy analysed for toxic metals. These would obviously be highly invasive and unpleasant tests that frankly wouldn't add much to your understanding.

The Problem with Tests

Tests have now come to be seen as some sort of objective 'gold standard' and override all other criteria such as taking a history, examination, signs and symptoms. They are not taken to be *a part* of the picture – they are assumed to *be* the picture. There are several problems with this approach.

The first concern is how samples were taken, stored and transported and how much time elapsed before testing could take place. Blood tests for the presence of circulating mercury, for instance, are thought to give off much of their mercury content as vapour in the first few hours and can be affected by the material used to store the sample.

No test is infallible and all tests are recognized to yield a proportion of both false negative and false positive results. This means that you might run a blood test for, say, cancer, and some people who actually have cancer would be told they were in the clear and some who do not have cancer would be told that they did. This is putting aside the human-error mix-ups that occasionally occur and the screening errors due to under-trained technicians.

Another issue is that because the medical profession does not understand FRS, they are fundamentally conducting meaningless tests. If you x-rayed your toaster because the fuse had gone, for instance, the test results would be negative. Another problem is that most tests will only answer the specific question(s) that the clinician asks. If no instructive results are obtained, it may just indicate that the wrong or irrelevant questions were asked. All tests, too, are a snapshot in time. So, the fact that your test might be normal today does not mean that it would have been normal yesterday or will be again tomorrow. There are particular problems inherent in thyroid function testing and these will be addressed in detail in chapter 10.

The Caring Professions

In spite of the fact that these syndromes have been officially recognized by committees of experts for decades, the notion still persists within the medical profession that they are all psychosomatic. This concept has gained ground partly because they don't understand what fatigue-related syndromes are, have no conclusive tests for them, don't have a pill to fix them and also because of outspoken 'experts' who insist that they are psychosomatic. Doctors buying in to this philosophy may prescribe antidepressants, cognitive behavioural therapy and graded exercise therapy (if they do anything at all) – all of which do nothing to address the underlying problem of toxicity.

Another issue is that many of these syndromes are 'invisible' and you most probably do not look as sick as you are. Don't forget that the doctor is, after all, used to seeing sick people all day and indeed the general population is unwell for much the same reasons as the FRS sufferer.

The term 'syndrome' refers to a collection of physical signs and symptoms such as insomnia or pain. Sometimes fatigue-related syndromes can have a big symptom picture, but be short on the signs – or the doctor may not know what signs to look for or how to elicit them.

You may be shocked to discover just how little sympathy or help you are offered, just when you are at your most vulnerable. Many sufferers experience being treated dismissively, abruptly or without compassion. In fact, two-thirds of CFS and fibromyalgia sufferers are actively unhappy with the treatment that they receive from allopathic medicine. Looking back now, I am not sure whether it would have been better or worse to have had an illness that the doctors thought they understood. If they had thought they understood the disease, they would probably have wanted to either operate or give me drugs. Neither of these options would have helped and both would have further delayed my search for effective help.

A History of Misadventure

It is worth remembering that some brutal and callous treatment has been meted out in less enlightened times. The mentally ill were frequently treated to inhumane therapies involving being stripped, chained up, dowsed in water, turned on a 'tranquilizing wheel' and subjected to sporadic bleedings by their physicians. Indeed the public could even buy tickets to watch this 'entertainment'. Expressions of sexual desire in females were considered to be a symptom of mental illness just over a century ago and were treated with clitoridectomy (surgical removal of the clitoris). The first cases of multiple sclerosis at the beginning of the 20th century were referred to in learned medical journals at the time as 'Faker's disease' and suggested treatments included a lashing! Lobotomies were used until as recently as 1970 to treat schizophrenia and we still use the cosh of electric shock treatment on something as delicate and complex as the brain to treat mental illness. The medical profession is often keen to dismiss conditions that they do not understand and, sadly, appear not to have learned any lessons from history.

The Desirable Patient

Doctors are only human and they like certain characteristics in an ideal patient. They prefer it if their clients are attractive (not necessarily good-looking, but personable and clean), and that they share common values. They also like the patient to have a complaint that is slightly interesting and/or challenging for them, but not something that demonstrates their ignorance. For this reason alone, medical personnel may feel uncomfortable and become hostile when confronted with a condition that they do not understand because, fundamentally, they can't help. A recent tragic case in the UK involved the alleged mercy killing of 31-year-old Lynn Gilderdale, who had CFS, by her mother who had been nursing her for 16 years. Having been an active teen, she had spent her adult life unable to swallow or move. As a consequence she was being tube-fed, had a host of disabling conditions, could not recognize or remember anything and was extremely sensitive to any sensory input. The verdict of the *specialist clinic* that was treating her was that she was an attention seeker with an invented illness! You may find yourself in the unenviable position of having to prove to doubting professionals that you are gravely and profoundly ill. Unfortunately, these same professionals act as the gatekeepers for benefits, sick notes and insurance claims which may mean that you struggle financially as well as physically.

Frankly, you probably haven't got long enough to wait for learned committees of medical experts to convene in conference rooms across the globe and to formally agree what causes the disease and what they can do about it. So even if you find an enlightened health professional who acknowledges that fatigue-related syndromes exist and that you have one, they still have no idea how to treat it, so it does not advance your cause.

Friends and Relatives

Because of the confusion surrounding this issue and because some very vocal doctors do not believe the condition exists at all, you may be shocked and surprised to find that you encounter hostility and disbelief. This may come from the very people – employers, colleagues, family and friends – whose support you require. Perversely, part of the problem is that people are used to sick people, and especially to relatively young sick people, recovering after an illness. So you may find that people are initially sympathetic, but then become bored by it all when you fail to improve over a period of months or years. By and large, others do not mean to be ignorant or cruel, they just don't understand – and you can't expect them to. Anyone who has never been seriously or chronically ill can have no comprehension of how you feel and the private, living hell of these conditions is known only to fellow FRS sufferers.

Work and Home

FRS may also bring other frustrations and pressures. The sufferer may not be able to work at all or may have to dramatically alter their ideas about the type or quantity of work that they can take on. A quarter of FRS sufferers are unable to work and may be on disability benefits and many more may have tried to make various claims and been denied. This can also incur the resentment of co-workers and partners and many have lost jobs, careers, scholarships, marriages and other relationships to the syndrome.

Many sufferers describe needing to do things for themselves in the times that they feel better, simply because there is no one else to delegate to. Many FRS sufferers are mothers with dependent children and they may not be capable of being the sort of mother they would like to be. They may not be able to take part in activities that others consider normal and may be emotionally drained and have no energy for fun. In fact, they may be struggling to cope at all. There may also be intimate relationships to consider with your partner and you may feel too sick or tired to be much fun or to feel like sex, which all takes its toll over time.

Chapter 6

Our Toxic Planet

And we have made of ourselves living cesspools, and
driven doctors to invent names for our diseases.

Plato

Hippocrates was stating a universal truth when he declared that 'All diseases are crises of purification, of toxic elimination,' 2,500 years ago. However, our bodies are now being challenged by toxins on a daily basis in a way that Hippocrates probably could not have imagined in his worst nightmares. This toxic overload is combined with a precipitous decline in the nutritional value of foods whereby the minerals and vitamins required to detoxify these substances are almost completely lacking in our diet. Many regard having two or three colds a year and regular headaches or indigestion as 'normal' and radiant good health accompanied by the ability to effectively combat infections as rare. In this chapter we examine the larger sources of toxicity, problems of deficiency and also some of the unseen environmental factors that contribute to FRS.

Toxins

Toxins are substances that have a detrimental effect on everyone and we are exposed to a perplexing array of them every minute of our lives. In the last 70 years, at least 75,000 new chemicals have been released into the environment, 93 per cent of which have *never been tested*. Three hundred of these are commonly found in our homes and 3,500 have been added to our food with the average child being exposed to 100mg (3.5oz) of chemicals every day. The blood of most adults and even babies tests positive to *at least 300 toxins*, many of which are highly synergistic. We also encounter toxic metals in general – and heavy metals in particular – routinely in a variety of seemingly innocent forms. As a result, the average adult now carries 700 times the levels of toxins of their forefathers! That is up to 3.5 kg (7.7lb) of toxins mostly stored in their body fat, joints and 'non-essential' body compartments such as the sinuses and uterus. These toxins harm us by interfering with our metabolic pathways, preventing our cells detoxifying and by disrupting our endocrine system.

In the history of mankind, we have never encountered such a massive toxic challenge and we are ill-equipped to deal with it. Many feel that by our actions we are currently conducting an uncontrolled mass experiment on the whole of humanity. The problem is that as our environment becomes ever more toxic, we necessarily become more toxic too. Whilst you cannot avoid exposure to many of these toxins, since they are found even in places as remote as the polar icecaps, you can substantially reduce your personal exposure to those that you consume, apply and inhale and this is addressed in chapter 16. A few of the modern-day toxins about which there is most concern are examined in more detail below.

Persistent Organic Pollutants (POPs)

DDT, polychlorinated biphenyl (PCB), dieldrin, polycyclic aromatic hydrocarbons (PAH) and some brominated flame retardants are all classified as persistent organic pollutants (POPs). These substances do not degrade and also bio-accumulate up the food chain, adversely affecting the environment and ultimately human health. Most of these chemicals have been, or are currently used as pesticides – although some are produced in industrial processes. The average adult is estimated to consume a gallon of pesticides and herbicides alone every year and these chemicals are highly synergistic. For example, a cocktail of three pesticides may produce 100 times the toxic effect of any one in isolation. Polybrominated diphenyl ethers (PBDE) are POPs which are widely used as flame-retardants and now contaminate salmon, dairy products and beef and are routinely identified in human breast milk. Perfluorinated chemicals (PFCs) in women have also been found to disrupt the menstrual cycle, affect fertility and impair the growth of the foetus.

Formaldehyde

Formaldehyde is widely used in the manufacture of plastics, foams, textiles, disinfectants, petroleum and pharmaceuticals, construction materials such as plywood, and in agriculture as a fumigant. The formaldehyde vapours are irritant, causing eye, skin, airway and lung irritation and are readily absorbed into the circulation via the lungs where they may cause headaches, depression and kidney damage.

Fluorine

Fluorine is rated as more poisonous than lead and only slightly less toxic than arsenic. It occurs naturally in tobacco and tea and is added to toothpaste, mouth rinses, used by dentists in dental gel and is added to some municipal water supplies. These supplies are fluoridated using small amounts (1 part per million) of fluoride waste product from either the aluminium or fertilizer processing industries in order to aid tooth-decay prevention. Whether it effectively prevents against decay or not, fluoride acquired from these and various additional sources results in fluorosis (an unsightly mottling of the teeth) and this may act as a 'window on the bones' where fluoride causes osteoporosis. Fluoride in toothpaste is routinely absorbed through the mucosa and gums and the amount of fluoride in a tube of toothpaste is enough to kill a small child. Symptoms of early skeletal fluorosis include many of the symptoms of FRS including muscle weakness and pains in the bones and joints, burning and tingling sensation in the limbs, tremors and cramps, premature ageing, digestive problems and chronic fatigue. Fluoride also adversely affects the immune system, inhibits testosterone and causes genetic damage and miscarriage. It particularly affects the parathyroid, thyroid and pineal glands by displacing essential elements such as iodine, binding other elements and interfering with enzyme systems. Accumulation of fluoride in the pineal gland diminishes the synthesis of melatonin, which is the most potent antioxidant to act within the brain, and may cause insomnia and precocious puberty. Fluoride also has a massive synergy with mercury and pesticides and enhances the absorption of lead.

Chlorine

The main source of chlorine is the tap water that we drink, use for cooking and washing food, and shower and bathe in. Our skin has a very large surface area and has been shown to readily absorb chlorine from bath and shower water, swimming pools, hot tubs and jacuzzis. When heated, chlorinated water gives off both a vapour and spray containing chloramine gas which can be inhaled and is also toxic. Chlorine is also used to bleach a lot of products including all paper, tampons, sanitary towels, toilet paper, cotton wool and even white foodstuffs such as sugar and flour. Other sources include antiseptics, household disinfectants and cleaners, bleach and Milton's solution. Most fruit and vegetables and all prepared salads are washed in chlorine solutions.

Both chlorine and fluorine are positively charged electrolytes that can react with almost any other chemical and combine in water to form trihalomethanes which are carcinogens that tend to be stored in the fatty tissues of the body. Chlorine is known to directly irritate the skin, lungs and eyes, to destroy the intestinal flora and to create massive oxidative tissue damage.

Radiation

Recent decades have seen the deployment and testing of the nuclear arsenal. This includes dozens of detonations in the western deserts of the US in the 1950s, over 200 tests by the French at the atolls of Polynesia and the nuclear bombs at Hiroshima and Nagasaki. More recently the disaster at Chernobyl and the use of depleted uranium shells in warfare have contributed to the radioactive contamination of the entire planet. This occurs as the winds carry radioactive particles that subsequently contaminate the soil. The use of x-rays for diagnosis and even the increased exposure to cosmic radiation at high altitudes from more frequent flying also contribute to a larger personal dose of ionizing radiation. The thyroid gland, in particular, appears to be especially vulnerable to damage from radiation.

We are our own guinea pigs.

Dr Roy E Albert

Deficiency

The average diet in the developed world is now low in fibre and high in over-processed, refined foods, salt, animal fats, sugar, insecticides, herbicides, pesticides, colourings, preservatives and stimulants such as caffeine and alcohol. Not only do these foods fail to nourish our bodies, but they act as 'anti-nutrients' in that they consume many minerals and vitamins in digestion and offer no nutritional value in return. Even when we do eat fruits and vegetables, they now have 50 per cent of the nutrients (on average) that they had just 50 years ago. Refine, cook, store, preserve or process these foods and these figures drop even more dramatically. Whilst many people are now vitamin deficient, almost everyone is deficient in one or more minerals. This is because we now use chemical fertilizers rather than the time-honoured methods of crop rotation and composting waste. These fertilizers also kill the symbiotic fungi which live on the roots of plants, aiding absorption of nutrients and especially minerals. These mineral-deficient soils necessarily mean mineral-deficient foods and ultimately mineral-deficient people.

Environmental Stressors

Another causative factor is that many FRS sufferers may unwittingly be living or working somewhere that is having a detrimental effect on their health. If this is the case, then no amount of effort to follow the advice in this book will be rewarded if you do not address these factors first. Geopathic and underground water stress are two categories of environmental stressors that relate primarily to natural phenomena occurring beneath the thin crust of the Earth that we inhabit. The third category, electromagnetic stress, refers to largely man-made emanations.

Geopathic Stress

Our planet has a giant magnetic core at its heart which creates an electromagnetic field that, when disturbed, can produce perturbations that have a detrimental effect on most living things. Disturbances can be caused either by naturally occurring formations such as geological faults, underground ore masses or cavities, or by man through nearby earthworks or mining, for instance. In Germany this is recognized and taken seriously and they refer to some towns with known geopathic stress issues as 'cancer towns'. No one is quite sure what the nature of the effect is, but differences in background gamma radiation have been detected in these areas. Geopathic stress may also be one of the factors behind 'sick-building syndrome', where office workers may take a lot of time off sick and never feel well in a particular office.

There are two grids of positive and negative electromagnetic energy lines covering the Earth's surface that are about 2 metres (6.5ft) apart. This means that, inevitably, some parts of your office or home will be affected by negative energy lines. The question is whether the places in which you spend a lot of time like your bed, desk, sofa or chair are situated on these lines. If you sleep poorly at home, but sleep better elsewhere, negative lines running through the area in which your bed is situated are a possibility. If you tend to feel unusually drained or tired after being in any specific location, try relocating the relevant sofa, desk or chair if possible. If you have a cat and it likes to sleep on your bed or sofa, that might indicate the presence of a negative energy line which appears to be beneficial to cats but detrimental to humans. However, if you own a dog which particularly likes to settle on your bed or sofa, you can be confident that they are on a positive energy line. Pests and weeds such as cockroaches, wasps' and ants' nests, mice, moss and moulds also favour negative energy lines.

Underground Water Stress

Because water conducts electricity so readily, underground water stress has a big impact on the electromagnetic field. This is the most damaging of the environmental stress categories and includes man-made sewers and drains and natural sudden changes in underground water levels within the Earth's crust.

Electromagnetic Stress

Although we consider it normal to live in brick houses with electricity cables and water pipes running through the walls, and nearby telephone masts and electricity pylons, there is nothing natural about it. Modern life all but demands the use of recently developed technologies such as digital and mobile phones, computers, televisions, microwave ovens and satellite navigation systems. All these devices generate both electrical and magnetic fields that are known to interfere with the proper functioning of the immune system and pineal gland and to cause oxidative damage. In fact, there is an almost certain link between EM radiation and leukemia, Alzheimer's disease and degenerative illness, and the World Health Organization has recently admitted that EM radiation is a possible carcinogen.

'Dirty' Electricity

A separate but related issue is that of so-called 'dirty' electricity. This refers to the surges of electromagnetic radiation that contaminate the normal power supply, or to the high-frequency voltage radiation that is generated when certain electrical appliances are used. This is known to be biologically active and has been particularly implicated in the causation of diabetes.

Early signs of EM sensitivity include eye problems such as smarting of the eyes and an aversion to light and then progress to some of the symptoms FRS sufferers are all too familiar with including depression, memory problems and weakness in the joints.

Other Negative Influences

Sometimes some places just have an uneasy energy that cannot be attributed to any of the above. Examples include the room in the house that never gets warm or that you or your pets don't like to dwell in for long or the occurrence of an occasional strange and unpleasant smell in certain locations. In these cases, you may want to consider calling in someone who specializes in dealing with such issues.

Chapter 7

The Symptoms of Fatigue-Related Syndromes and Their Causes

This chapter addresses the main symptoms of fatigue-related syndromes and examines their likely causes. Almost all of the factors cited elsewhere as risk factors such as depression, digestive problems and sleep disturbance are probably *early onset symptoms* and can predate the diagnosis of full-blown FRS by several decades. All body systems and organs are affected in FRS to a greater or lesser degree and different symptoms may come to the fore for an hour, a day, a week or a month. This can be frustrating and confusing for the sufferer, and can add to the notion in others' minds that these symptoms are imagined.

Being Female

Female FRS sufferers outnumber male sufferers by nine to one. This, in itself, presents a problem where the male-dominated medical profession may not be able to empathize with or take 'women's problems' as seriously as they do those of men. Most women will have taken synthetic sex hormones either as the pill or as HRT at some stage, had one or more babies with all the care and nutrient depletion that involves and then may also have experienced the final hormonal challenge unique to women: the menopause. Broadly speaking, women are still regarded as second-class citizens and are also expected to be dutiful and 'nice', with a lot of feelings consequently being repressed from an early age. Factor in having more vaccinations, dental treatment and antibiotics, possible yo-yo dieting that may have stressed the entire endocrine system and the fact that women accumulate mercury at twice the rate of men and it is perhaps not such a surprising finding after all!

Stress and Trauma

Sometimes the onset of FRS is triggered by a final or overwhelming insult such as an infection, exposure to an allergen or toxin, a vaccination, a car accident, a house move, a divorce or bankruptcy. The term 'stress' is generally used fairly loosely, but the medical use of the word denotes anything that the body has to mount a response to. On a very mundane level being cold, having an infection or poorly controlled blood sugar levels are all significant stressors to which the body has to respond. Then there are the kinds of stresses most would recognize such as being bullied at work, moving house, bereavement, redundancy, divorce or separation. The personality profile of a typical FRS sufferer is of someone who is ambitious, hard-working and perfectionistic and who expects a lot of themselves and others. In this manner, a lot of the stress experienced may have been self-induced. Typically, sufferers may also have been 'running on empty' for a long time, possibly living on stimulants such as coffee, chocolate, sugar and cigarettes and possibly having an inadequate or poor diet before the point of no return is unwittingly passed.

Childhood Stress

Although FRS sufferers respond poorly to stress and may have been under pressure in the run-up to becoming ill, critically they may also have experienced an unusual amount of stress as a child. This may have taken the form of the death of a parent, sexual or physical abuse or experiencing a life-threatening illness or accident. On a slightly more mundane level, being sent away to boarding school or to live with relatives, being bullied or general family instability all set the stage for later illness. The specific mechanisms by which this occurs are discussed in detail in chapter 11.

Vaccinations

The vaccination programme may generally have a detrimental effect on the immune system as a result of the cumulative effect of the number of toxic insults. Alternatively, a particular vaccination may be the straw that breaks the camel's back and sufferers can often date the advent of their FRS to a recent vaccination. This topic is addressed in chapter 8.

Fatigue

Fatigue has come to be a very common complaint and is not at all normal, although we have come to regard it as such. The central presenting symptom of FRS is a profound and persistent physical and mental fatigue that borders on exhaustion and that is not relieved – or is only partially relieved – by rest. Also typically there is a 'post-exertional malaise' which refers to a worsening of symptoms and a pathologically slow recovery period after exertion. One explanation for this finding relates to the poisoning of the mitochondria and this is covered in more detail in chapter 9.

Musculoskeletal Dysfunction

The pain experienced in FRS is usually widespread and migratory in nature and includes a significant degree of muscle and/or joint pain. Typically this pain centres on the shoulder, back and/or neck region and there is also a high incidence of chronic pelvic pain. It may be that the muscles in these regions work the hardest and so are the worst affected. It is also possible that during pubertal growth of the pelvis toxins may have been incorporated there and whilst this may result in pain and stiffness, it is not life threatening. Alternatively, the osteopath and founder of kinesiology, Dr George Goodheart, discovered that all the muscles are associated with specific organ systems. The muscles of the neck and shoulder relate to the stomach, brain, immune system, kidney and bladder, whereas those controlling the hips relate to the kidneys, sex hormones and large intestine. The kidneys are profoundly and adversely affected by metal toxicity and this causes the related psoas and iliacus muscles (which run internally within the pelvis) to become hypertonic (spasm). Metal toxicity also progressively compromises the other systems listed and this may account for the intractable nature of the hip and shoulder pain. The bladder, too, is impacted by toxic metals and the bladder meridian runs over both the shoulders and the entire length of the spine (see figure 47), and distress of this internal organ may manifest in neck, back and shoulder pain. The migratory nature of the pain is due to the fact that according to Traditional Chinese Medicine the body is always moving its toxic burden around according to the time of day – a bit like tankers carrying a toxic cargo that no country wants.

There are also relationships between where symptoms appear and emotional issues. The upper back relates to stress and lack of emotional support; the shoulders to the burdens we carry; the neck to the ability to look at the past and the hips to the ability to move forwards in life.

Temperomandibular Joint Dysfunction

Temperomandibular joint dysfunction (TMD or TMJ) is often found in FRS and is the term used when there is a problem with the articulation of the mandible (jaw bone) within its socket on the base of the skull in the temporal bone. This joint may click or lock and does not permit the smooth opening and closing of the mouth and this can cause pain in the temples, jaw and face. The sensory input from the temperomandibular joint accounts for nearly half of the total input from the body, so it must be very important to have been biologically prioritized in this way. Several possible explanations have been proposed including a structural compensation for pelvic or sphenoid problems (a bone in the base of the brain), infection with Chlamydia trachomatis, historic trauma causing a protective muscular bracing, and repressed anger. In Chinese Medicine, the muscles that control the jaw are related to the kidneys and adrenal glands and the meridians which relate to the digestive and endocrine systems also run over this region. Finally, being close to the source, mercury toxicity may particularly affect both the controlling trigeminal nerves and the jaw joints.

Pain

In addition to the muscle and joint pain commonly experienced, some FRS sufferers also find that they experience headaches that are new in type, severity or duration, bone, eye, nerve or testicular pain, and painful skin sensitivity. Toxicity of the reticular activating system which is known to modulate experience of pain within the body may be responsible for causing this enhanced perception of pain, as may toxicity of the affected body parts.

Sleep Dysfunction

This, again, may be an early sign of FRS, but may also be a causative factor. Sleep may initially be disrupted by extrinsic factors such as shift work or jet lag, chronic diseases such as bronchitis, pain, caring for babies or children, sleep apnoea (ceasing to breathe during sleep), or taking certain prescription drugs. Many FRS sufferers may find that needing to urinate frequently in the night disrupts sleep too.

Once the syndrome is established, common findings include unrefreshing, poor sleep, insomnia, sleep/wake cycle disturbances, nightmares, vivid and disturbing dreams, or sleeping the sleep of the dead and waking feeling awful. The normal rhythms and patterns of sleep are also altered and in contrast to healthy people, exercise can also worsen the sleep dysfunction. This symptom is most probably a direct consequence of mercury toxicity affecting the controlling glands in the brain that regulate sleep/wake cycles and sleep induction.

Pharmaceutical and Recreational Drug Use

You may be surprised to see pharmaceutical drugs (both over-the-counter and prescription) being categorized with recreational drugs. As far as your body is concerned, however, there is not a great deal of difference because all drugs are toxic and all have some unwelcome side effects. The only difference is that recreational drugs have direct effects on the central nervous system that are experienced as being pleasant. Recent research seems to indicate that as little as one exposure to cannabis can cause life-long alterations in brain chemistry that can later manifest as depression, bipolar disorder and psychosis. The body chemistry is in a very fragile state of balance and can easily be thrown off course by these exogenous substances. The effects of particular pharmaceuticals are discussed in chapter 16.

Respiratory Problems

Many FRS sufferers experience some kind of difficulty breathing including frequent, shallow breathing, perceived difficulty or pain on breathing, a chronic cough, shortness of breath, or sleep apnoea. This may be because the vast majority of mercury is absorbed as vapour in the lungs and this, when combined with toxicity of the hypothalamus, compromises the autonomic regulation of breathing.

Hypoglycaemia

Problems with poorly controlled blood sugar, too, are thought to precipitate FRS, but are probably an early manifestation of the syndrome. This may occur for several reasons. First, our modern diets of refined and sugar-laden foods cause blood sugar challenges that the body struggles to respond to. Second, glucose tolerance factor (GTF), which aids blood sugar control and utilization of glucose by the cells, requires the trace mineral, chromium, and this may be deficient in the diet or poorly absorbed. Third, pancreatic function is adversely affected by the presence of toxic metals – especially arsenic – and also by endocrine dysfunction. Toxic metals also bind to the insulin receptor sites on the cells rendering the circulating hormone ineffective and creating insulin resistance which is a pre-diabetic state. Finally, the pancreas can be detrimentally affected by 'dirty' electricity and emotional issues such as having lost a child or being separated from your mother and this latter topic is discussed in more detail in chapter 10.

Weight Change

Without significant changes in diet, unexplained weight gain or weight loss may both be found. Weight loss may be a function of poor digestion, a parasitic infection, an overactive thyroid gland, dysfunctional hypothalamus and/or pituitary glands, diabetes or pre-diabetes, coeliac disease, or adrenal exhaustion. The most common cause of weight gain probably relates to an underactive thyroid gland or a dysfunctional hypo-thalamus and/or pituitary gland, but eating foods to which you are intolerant is also a significant cause. The body may also carry stubborn excess water or fat in an effort to dilute or store noxious substances. Unfortunately, as visceral fat collects around the organs it produces oestrogen which encourages further fat deposition, antagonizes thyroxine and suppresses the immune system. It also puts pressure on the intestine, thus compromising blood flow and creating a vicious cycle which promotes damage to the intestinal lining.

Digestive Deficiencies

The digestive system is one of the first systems to be affected in FRS and symptoms such as nausea, IBS, diarrhoea, constipation, abdominal pain, bloating, an urgent need to defecate with occasional loss of continence, excessive flatulence and 'wet wind' may predate the diagnosis of FRS by several decades. In fact, nearly 90 per cent of US females have occasional digestive problems with *70 per cent being affected every day*, so this is a massive and growing issue. Swallowed mercury is absorbed directly into the massive plexus of autonomic nerves that control all the processes of digestion and results in a progressive decline in production of all digestive enzymes and compromised peristal-sis. The hypothalamus too may be directly affected by mercury vapour and this controls the vagus nerve and the autonomic regulation of the organs of digestion. The presence of mercury in the intestine also blocks the action of protease enzymes in general and in particular those that digest the relatively large molecules in gluten (in wheat, rye, barley and oats) and casein (in dairy products). The combination of undigested food and mercury toxicity in the intestines also creates an ideal environment for overgrowth of the yeast Candida albicans as discussed in chapter 8.

Liver and Gall Bladder Dysfunction

The liver is always seriously compromised in all chronic disease and the gall bladder is invariably affected because the toxic bile is further concentrated there. The bile is green because it contains some of the breakdown products of haemoglobin from the red blood cells, but colours the faeces brown. Poor or erratic function of the gall bladder means that the faeces can vary from a very pale clay colour (no bile and full of fat), through various yellow ochre colours to green. When the gall bladder is not functioning properly the food particles become covered in fat which means that the enzymes that break down proteins and carbohydrates are ineffective. This causes fermentation and production of gas in the large intestine, the stool may be greasy and float due to the fat content, and undigested food may clearly be evident.

Nutritional Deficiencies

Nutritionally poor diets, especially those high in carbohydrates and low in protein, may have a role in initiating and perpetuating FRS. Vegan and vegetarian diets are often low in the proteins required to detoxify toxic metals and to repair and build tissue. Deficiencies of specific nutrients – due to a poor diet or poor absorption – such as vitamin B12 or vitamin D, essential fatty acids or minerals such as iron or magnesium are also thought to be predisposing factors. The topics of diet and supplementation for FRS are addressed in detail in chapters 14 and 17 respectively.

Endocrine Dysfunction

The endocrine organs often preferentially accumulate mercury because they are very metabolically active, have a high fat content and contain a lot of mineral receptors that attract and bind toxic metals. Whilst the system can compensate for primary dysfunction in a specific gland in the short term, ultimately the whole endocrine system is compromised to the level of function of the worst-affected organ. Disorders of the thyroid gland are the most commonly identified, with disorders of the adrenal glands (leading to poor stress response), the pancreas (leading to poor blood sugar control), and the testes or ovaries (leading to reproductive or sexual dysfunction) also commonly occurring. The hypothalamus regulates the endocrine response and is vulnerable to mercury vapour from amalgam fillings and this may create potentially lifelong endocrine dysfunction. These issues are discussed in further detail in chapter 10.

Low Body Temperature

A low core body temperature may be a result of dysfunction of the hypothalamus, the inability to generate heat because of the compromised function of the liver (the main heat-generating organ) and/or a low metabolic rate. Many also experience cold hands and feet which may be due to the body storing toxins in the extremities and then reducing the circulation to these areas. Conversely, many FRS sufferers also find heat uncomfortable since they cannot disperse it through the skin because the circulation is so compromised.

Viral and Bacterial Infections

The immune system is one of the early casualties of FRS and this means that the body can no longer effectively control the microbes that it encounters. Yeasts can flourish and viruses and some bacteria can 'hide' within cells unchecked by the immune system and attempts to destroy them give rise to the appearance of autoimmunity. The hypothalamus also orchestrates immunity and may also be responsible for a compromised immune response. The result of all this is chronic and recurrent infections, tender enlarged lymph nodes in the neck, armpit and groin, and a persistent sore throat because of swollen tonsils and/or adenoids. Early removal of either the adenoids or tonsils appears to be associated with FRS and this may be because important defences have been removed or because lymphatic drainage of the head and neck has been compromised by scar tissue. Alternatively, the same agent(s) may be responsible for both the inflammation of these glands and ultimately for producing the FRS.

Sometimes an acute viral or bacterial infection can tip a seemingly healthy individual into an FRS and this is discussed in more detail in chapter 8.

Candidiasis

Overgrowth of the yeast Candida albicans, is an almost universal finding in FRS. It is the result of mercury toxicity, a poor immune system, a compromised digestive system and a refined diet, and is aided and abetted by the use of pharmaceuticals such as antibiotics and the contraceptive pill. Under these conditions it can change into its mycelial fungal form and perforate the intestines causing a 'leaky gut'. This permits the release of candotoxins, yeast spores and also improperly digested foods into the circulation, causing the individual to feel unwell, develop a systemic yeast infection and food intolerances. This subject is explored in greater detail in chapter 8.

Alcohol Intolerance

Since yeast overgrowth is almost invariably a problem in FRS, the sufferer may have been producing endogenous alcohol for decades. This means that the associated liver detoxification pathways are overloaded and as a consequence, alcohol intolerance is a common finding. This is also discussed further in chapter 14.

Allergies and Intolerances

The development of a leaky gut combined with an immune system which is overwhelmed by toxic metals, pathogens and their toxins and improperly digested food molecules, can become overactive, underactive or just plain confused. As the detoxification pathways in the liver are overwhelmed and the immune system becomes progressively more dysfunctional, the individual may develop more and more sensitivities to foods and chemicals. Mercury toxicity also unfavourably alters the ratios of T lymphocytes which promote, but may fail to terminate an immune response leading to the development of allergies.

Lymphatic Dysfunction

Mercury, being particularly lipophilic (fat-loving) accumulates in the lymphatic tissue. Here, the autonomic pumping of the lymphatic vessels may be compromised, leading to stagnation of the lymph and symptoms such as swelling of the ankles. Sometimes individuals can feel more comfortable with their arms raised over their head (without realizing why), because this position better facilitates drainage of the lymph into the general circulation. Clenching and grinding of the teeth (often at night) may also be a desperate attempt by the body to circulate stagnant lymph.

Autoimmunity

In autoimmunity, the body seemingly attacks its own cells which it mistakes as 'non-self' and there is often a family history of autoimmune diseases in those with FRS. There may be no such entity as 'autoimmune disease' *per se*, but two possibilities exist. The first is that mercury attaches to the 'self' coding on the cell membrane, changing it so that it is read by the immune system as 'non-self'. The appearance of heredity probably relates to a familial lack of enzymes for detoxification pathways or a particularly high requirement for a specific nutrient. The second possibility is that the immune system persistently attempts to root out latent viruses and other infective agents within the cells which may give rise to the appearance of autoimmunity. The reaction to all this is usually to prescribe steroids which further compromises any effective response. The emotional significance of autoimmunity may literally relate to self-hatred or 'attacking the self'.

Urinary Dysfunction

Many FRS sufferers may also need to urinate frequently or may experience occasional urinary incontinence or stress incontinence (leakage of urine when laughing, sneezing or running). The bladder is an early casualty of metal toxicity (which may manifest as 'cystitis') and over time the autonomic control of the bladder and associated sphincters diminishes, compromising bladder control.

Reproductive Dysfunction

Female sufferers of FRS frequently have a history of endometriosis, miscarriage, infertility, an irregular and painful menstrual cycle, heavy menstrual bleeding, ovarian cysts, hysterectomy, breast tenderness and PMS. Males may have lowered sperm counts or ineffective sperm. In women, the body tends to store toxins in the uterus and the sensitive processes of egg formation (in females) and sperm production (in males) are easily perturbed by toxic metals and other toxins. The hypothalamus also regulates both ovarian and testicular function and toxicity of this gland may also be involved in producing reproductive mayhem.

Sexual Dysfunction

This, too, is a very 'normal' part of FRS with greatly reduced sexual sensitivity and responsiveness, and loss of libido. Male sufferers may be unable to achieve or maintain an erection and both sexes are likely to experience difficulties with arousal or orgasm, with some female sufferers also complaining of vulval pain or pain on intercourse. The hypothalamus controls sexual behaviour and toxicity of this gland may ultimately be responsible for these issues. There may also be a history of traumatic abortions, miscarriages or birth experiences in women, and both sexes may have experienced sexual abuse, rape, sexual rejection or betrayal which may inform the condition.

Central Nervous System Dysfunction

Mercury is a potent neurotoxin which tracks up the nerves into the brain and spinal cord and this creates a sort of toxic one-way system. In this way, toxic metals progressively accumulate in the central nervous system whilst being afforded the extra protection offered to these precious organs. This is the normally irreversible mechanism at work in other conditions such as Parkinson's disease, multiple sclerosis and Alzheimer's disease. The effects of mercury on the brain have been referred to as a 'partial chemical lobotomy' and this may account for the profound structural and functional degenerative changes revealed by the imaging of FRS sufferers' brains.

As a result, FRS sufferers typically experience difficulties with cognitive function such as poor concentration and memory, difficulty making decisions and retrieving words and names, anxiety, forgetfulness, mental fatigue, confusion and disorientation. The hypothalamus produces chemicals that promote learning and memory, and toxicity of this gland may also help to account for some of these symptoms. Two 2009 papers showed that the later development of Alzheimer's disease was associated with poor memory in mid-life and since both FRS and Alzheimer's are primarily caused by toxicity of the central nervous system, this is not a surprising finding. In addition, the FRS sufferer can have difficulty comprehending auditory information, become sensitive to loud noises and bright lights and easily become overwhelmed. This finding may be because the reticular activating system which should filter the passage of information into conscious awareness is adversely affected by toxicity.

Depression

The term 'psychosomatic' is an allopathic concept that relates to illnesses that affect the body but originate in the mind. This idea arose because of the construction of an artificial separation between psychic (psychiatric) and somatic (physical) illnesses. However, the brain is an organ and part of the body too and any abnormality that produces symptoms in the body will produce symptoms in the brain and vice versa. The majority of FRS sufferers have had a major depressive illness and half have experienced a major depressive episode. This depression is then assumed to be the *cause* of the physical illness, hence the label 'psychosomatic'. However, the depression that FRS sufferers experience contrasts with primary depression in that the MRI scans reveal notable structural differences, motivation is still present and the depression is not improved by exercise. The depression associated with FRS largely relates to mercury toxicity of the central nervous system and specifically toxicity of the pituitary gland. Mercury is known to reduce production of the feel-good hormone, oxytocin, from the pituitary and also to derange lithium metabolism which is known to protect and stabilize the nervous system. This form of depression may specifically induce a death wish or suicidal thoughts and will be resolved by effective detoxification.

Lack of Coordination

The cerebellum is a separate part of the brain adjacent to where the spinal cord and the thinking brain (cerebrum) meet and it is responsible for muscular coordination and control. Toxicity or compromised oxygen supply of the cerebellum and the hippocampus (which is part of the limbic system in the brain) can cause poor coordination (e.g. difficulty writing), misjudgement of distances and unsteadiness and clumsiness.

Cardiovascular Dysfunction
Blood Pressure

Many FRS sufferers have low blood pressure and postural hypotension, meaning that they often feel dizzy or faint on standing. In a healthy person, the autonomic nervous system and adrenaline (epinephrine) combine to constrict the blood vessels of the torso to prevent blood from pooling in the legs. In the FRS sufferer, however, both these responses are compromised, leading to a delayed and inadequate response. This creates a temporary deficit to the brain whilst allowing blood to pool in the rectum (causing haemorrhoids) and in the legs (causing varicose veins). Toxicity of the reticular activating system (which controls heart rate) and the hypothalamus (which controls blood pressure) may also be responsible for the finding of low blood pressure.

Palpitations

Several possible mechanisms may account for the palpitations some FRS sufferers experience. First, the cells of the heart have an inherent rhythm which is usually overridden by the ANS (autonomic nervous system) and it may be that this regulation is dysfunctional. Alternatively or additionally, mercury is known to preferentially accumulate in the heart and to interfere with the enzyme systems involved in heart contractions causing dysregulation. Some may also experience a racing, hammering heartbeat that can be sustained over a period of hours after eating foods to which they are intolerant or due to improperly digested food in circulation as a result of a 'leaky gut'. Finally, eating or drinking food containing excitotoxins such as aspartame or monosodium glutamate (MSG) is another possible cause.

Skin Conditions

The skin may become very pale and thin with pronounced facial pallor when tired. Alternatively, it may take on a yellow tinge due to poor liver function and this can make the skin itchy and cause sweaty, smelly feet. Some sufferers may have marked dark circles under their eyes and this variously can be attributed to kidney, adrenal or liver dysfunction. Frequent bouts of acne may also be experienced which may either be an attempt to detoxify through the skin, a result of poorly controlled blood sugar levels or adrenal exhaustion. Other common symptoms include red, mottled skin, spontaneous bruising, and crawling and stabbing skin sensations and tingling. The soles of the feet and the palms of the hands are particularly affected in hypothyroidism and can become highly coloured with dry, cracked skin especially on the heels and dry, splitting fingernails which lack half-moons and have fragile cuticles.

Wherever mercury is stored, overgrowth of Candida inevitably follows and as a result, many FRS sufferers experience persistent athlete's foot, or fungal finger- or toenails. The Candida is systemic (in your body) and particularly affects the extremities, and when the feet get hot and damp the Candida has a chance to grow. The same mechanism is at work in vaginal thrush, 'jock itch' and in skin creases and folds such as the crotch, belly (if overweight with an 'apron' of fat) and under the breasts. This is the body's way of trying to eject the Candida through the skin.

Many FRS sufferers experience some hair loss, especially of underarm or pubic hair, but may lose hair from their head and men, in particular, may lose hair from their lower leg. Common causes of alopecia include adrenal exhaustion, a parasitic infection, the presence of toxic metals (especially mercury), iodide deficiency and an underactive thyroid gland. Mercury toxicity has also been associated with greying hair.

Ear Disorders

Various ear problems such as deafness, earaches, vertigo, dizziness, recurrent ear infections, distorted hearing and tinnitus are all common findings. The cavities of the ear are a common site for storage of toxic metals and, as a result, Candida and other infections. The tubal tonsil which permits drainage of the middle ear can be adversely affected by metal toxicity with the result that there is a build-up of toxic lymph that causes so-called 'glue ear'. Other ear problems are probably the direct result of metal toxicity on autonomic nerves serving the ear and organs of balance. Ear problems are also commonly found in hypothyroidism possibly for the same reasons.

Eye Disorders

Some sort of deterioration of the eyes and eyesight is not uncommon, but is accepted by the population at large as being an inevitable part of ageing. Astigmatism, near-sightedness and dry and/or painful eyes are all common findings. Also found are visual disturbances such as blurry vision, 'floaters' (drifting dark patches within the eye), tunnel vision and blind spots. An inability to focus, prescription changes throughout the course of the day and sensitivity to oncoming headlights when driving also commonly occur. Again, the eyes provide relatively safe storage for toxins and the autonomic nervous supply which controls focusing is adversely and almost universally affected over time by toxicity.

The Mouth

Some FRS sufferers experience a dry mouth and many have a bright red colouration of the membranes at the back of the throat. This typically occurs next to the molar teeth and worsens with deterioration in symptoms and fades with improvement. Could it be possible that this is an indication that the source of the problem is in the mouth? Some denture wearers in particular may also experience persistent problems with oral thrush as described above.

Chapter 8
Living Matter

Most allopathic and holistic therapists alike, when presented with an individual's infection, will seek to eradicate it using either pharmaceuticals or natural compounds. I know both as a therapist and as a sufferer that this approach has little long-term value (although it may be necessary on occasions) and that invariably the 'infection' returns. So what if our fundamental assumptions on this topic are completely wrong? The paradigm that I outline below is most probably a complete reversal of everything that you think you know about infections. It also requires that we trace the roots of this approach back to their inception with Louis Pasteur in 19th-century Paris.

Germ Theory

Pasteur posited that germs could only exist in *one form* (monomorphism) and that they attacked the organism from *without*. This is the military model of infection which gives rise to the wish to defend oneself from these invasions and also to the notion that killing the 'enemy' microbe will restore order. Since the release of Pasteur's documents (which he specifically requested remain secret for a hundred years after his death), it has become evident that much of his research was not as claimed at the time. He famously recanted on his deathbed, but by then his deceptions had earned him and his theory the pre-eminent place in history he had probably wanted. Pasteur's Parisian contemporary and rival, Antoine Beauchamp, had proposed a competing theory (which was eclipsed by Pasteur's germ theory) he called pleomorphism. In it he maintained that microbes can take a *variety of different forms* and are generated *within* the individual from granules in the blood and cells (which are clearly visible in live specimens) in response to changes in the terrain. His work was later confirmed by many others, including Dr Günther Enderlein, who identified the granules as being micro-organisms that he called 'endobionts'. Dr Enderlein observed that under increasingly acidic conditions, these endobionts morphed first into bacteria, then fungi and finally, under extreme conditions, into viruses. In those who primarily eat a natural diet high in fruits and vegetables alkaline conditions will prevail, whereas the modern diet of refined and processed foods is acid-forming. The endobionts' ultimate function is to serve as an inbuilt mechanism that biodegrades living matter and returns it to the soil from which it arose. This theory may also explain why microbes possess such sophisticated means of controlling their host's behaviour using small molecules (which are often toxic) to communicate with the host's brain.

> **Infection is no war in which the body is fighting invaders. The bacteria that come to these sites are symbiotic and help the body in elaborating dead cells and tissue for expulsion. Infection … is a body cleaning process for a body burdened with toxic materials.**
>
> **T C Fry**

There is obviously enough truth in Pasteur's theory for it to have survived over a hundred years and whilst bacteria and viruses may be infective once generated they also require a hospitable terrain in which to multiply. This explains why some people do not catch colds or even HIV when exposed to the causative agents and why some survived the great plagues that claimed so many lives. This also accounts for why most people test positive to most microbes. The organisms responsible for MRSA and meningitis, for instance, are both commonly found, so why do they become such potent pathogens in some and yet appear to co-habit perfectly well in others?

To advance this theory further, what if this mechanism is nature's way of dealing with pathology? What if the microbe, rather than being our foe, is our greatest ally? When all potential detoxification routes are overwhelmed, causing toxins to back up in the tissues, is it possible that these organisms are generated in order to clean up or bind these toxic wastes to prevent them harming the individual? This may only be intended as a temporary measure until the processes of detoxification can resume. However, if no such reversal is ever forthcoming, is it then possible that parasite eggs (to which we are all constantly exposed) may develop in this compromised system in order to further bind and engulf the microbes?

Using any method – allopathic or holistic – to kill microbes and parasites is a 'germ theory' approach and is treating a symptom rather than a cause. It can also be counter-productive because the microbes or parasites release their cargo of toxic metals in addition to many other noxious breakdown products. Heavy overgrowth of any microbe then is a response to toxicity and the amount of necrotic tissue being generated. The pathologists in Mozart's Vienna were apparently all too familiar with the grey organs in the bodies of those who had died of mercury poisoning. Can you imagine how compromised the circulation must have been and how much necrotic tissue, toxicity and fungal overgrowth there has to be before organs actually become *grey*? The endobionts have effectively been signalled to start their job of decomposition whilst these unfortunate individuals were still alive and this may be the process at work in FRS!

Unlike bacteria and yeasts, viruses are not regarded as living, because they are just genetic material in a protective outer shell with an injecting mechanism. They function by inserting their genome into the host's cells and in this manner can control the cell's functions and use the cell to replicate.

> **What hope is there for medical science to ever become a true science when the entire structure of medical knowledge is built around the idea that there is an entity called disease which can be expelled when the right drug is found?**
>
> **Dr John H Tilden, MD**

The Appearance of Infectivity

There are several possibilities that might account for the *appearance* of infectivity.

- The first is that we all collectively become vulnerable through vitamin D deficiency as we head into the winter months.
- The second is that with toxicity comes cell death and the dismantling of the cell's components for recycling (known as apoptosis). Viruses may be the fragments of genetic material that are being packaged for transport and not *the cause* of the destruction.
- Another theory relates to the fact that we are all passengers on a planet hurtling through space at unimaginable speeds. On our adventures in outer space we travel through photon bands and are subject to local changes in background electrical and magnetic radiation. This is in addition to the daily, monthly, seasonal and annual cycles we are all familiar with, the solar flares and sunspots generated in our own solar system and the changes in barometric and atmospheric conditions that occur with changes of weather. Epidemics have a history of burning around the globe and then dying out – often against a background of deprivation as with the great flu epidemic at the end of the First World War. These may be generated in some way we don't fully understand by the global conditions to which we are all exposed. This may be allied to the theory that viruses may have 'hitched a ride' in our DNA for one or more generations and are actually being *expelled* from the cell under certain atmospheric conditions.

So in summary, it is man-made toxicity that is the problem and not nature, which is working in our best interests at all times. Of course, we have only polluted our bodies with the same careless disregard that we have shown our host planet and in a holographic universe how could it not be thus?

The part can never be well unless the whole is well.

Plato

Chronic and Recurrent Infections

For the reasons outlined above and because the delicate mechanisms of the immune system have been poisoned, chronic and recurrent infections are a universal issue in FRS. In the following section, we examine the various microbes and parasites that are frequently associated with the failing health of FRS. However, focusing on the particular 'infective' organism rather than on changing the terrain to encourage a more normal ecology might be a giant allopathic germ theory 'red herring'!

Bacterial Infections

The bacteria associated with salmonella, pneumonia, chlamydia and tuberculosis and a particular subset of bacteria known as mycoplasma are all suspected of involvement in FRS. However, by far the most important bacteria is Borrelia burgdorferi which is associated with Lyme disease or borreliosis, and we examine this in detail below.

Lyme Disease

Lyme borreliosis is a spirochete infection contracted from a tick bite in much the same way as malaria is transmitted by mosquitoes. Deer, cows, sheep, cats, birds and rodents can all carry these ticks, which, possibly because of global warming appear to be flourishing and now inhabit areas that previously did not pose a problem. The initiating tick bite will induce an angry rash, but for many FRS sufferers this event is lost in the mists of time. In the early stages the individual may have headaches and flu-like symptoms, but the disease can then progress to affect almost any body system and mimics other infections, for which Lyme disease has earned the title 'the great imitator'. Secondary sites of infection can cause muscle and joint pains, arthritis, heart abnormalities, neurological and psychiatric complaints and/or profound fatigue. Although the initial infection is probably contracted via a tick bite, it seems to be possible for the disease to be passed to intimate family members and certainly from mother to child through the placenta. Lyme disease is one of the fastest-growing infectious diseases and whilst it seems to be carried by a majority of people, it often finds a hospitable environment in those suffering with mercury toxicity. The ubiquitous staphylococcus is closely related to borrelia and it may also be that the body does not mount an effective response to borrelia, mistaking it for its less aggressive and more familiar cousin. Antibiotics are ineffective against borrelia and this may be because the heavy metals that encourage growth of these bacteria also deactivate the antibiotics deployed against them.

Fungal Infections

Fungi propagate by releasing spores (their yeast form) which, when they settle upon a suitable substrate can grow into their filamentous mould or fungal form. There are several fungi that are associated with FRS including various members of the Candida family. Although fungi reproduce asexually (usually resulting in identical 'copies'), Candida has developed a means of changing its genes dynamically in response to its environment and so has created a huge family tree. Several members of the Candida and Aspergillus families of moulds have been implicated in FRS, however Candida albicans is widely regarded as being the most common fungal infection found in FRS and is examined in detail below.

Overgrowth of Candida Albicans

> **Candida: It may not kill you, but it will take your life.**
>
> **David Newman**

Candida albicans is a commensal yeast that is found practically universally on skin and in the intestines. Its growth is normally checked by the 500 other organisms it cohabits the intestines with and is ultimately controlled by the immune system. However, in recent decades candidal overgrowth has become an increasing issue with many people exhibiting persistent and very resistant overgrowth of this yeast. Women tend to suffer from candidiasis more than men and this may be because oestrogen encourages the growth of Candida.

There may be many factors that contribute to candidal overgrowth including:

- The almost universal exposure to antibiotics which kill all the endogenous 'friendly' bacteria, thus removing one of the main factors controlling the spread of Candida.
- Drinking chlorinated water and the use of preservatives in foods which, in addition to killing any pathogens, also kill the friendly bacteria in the intestines.

- The use of steroid drugs such as asthma inhalers, corticosteroid creams, the contraceptive pill and HRT which suppress the immune response.
- A diet deficient in fruits and vegetables and rich in sugars, dairy, refined carbohydrates and yeast-containing foods which promote overgrowth of Candida.
- The use of pharmaceuticals – especially ulcer drugs, tranquillizers, sleeping pills and antacids and the frequent use of over-the-counter medication such as painkillers and any recreational drugs.
- Chronic stress, which raises blood sugar levels and depresses the immune system.

However, the single biggest reason for epidemic overgrowth of Candida albicans relates to the use of mercury in dental amalgam and we will examine this in more detail below. Candida is able to convert mercury from one form to another and also to generate energy in the process. The immune system is also adversely affected by the

Figure 2: The symptoms of candidiasis

Body System	Symptoms
Digestive system	Heartburn; indigestion; constipation; bloating; diarrhoea; continuous dull abdominal ache; food sensitivities; an urgent need to defecate and flatulence.
Genito-urinary system	Inflammation of the prostate gland; vaginal thrush; PMT; endometriosis; cystitis and the need for frequent urination.
Respiratory system	Bronchitis; asthma; recurrent chest infections and exaggerated reactions to other inhaled allergens including hay fever.
Nervous system	Impaired memory; confusion; mood swings; irritability; depression and loss of libido.
Ear, nose and throat	Recurrent ear, nose, throat and sinus infections; sensitivity to tobacco smoke.
Musculoskeletal system	Joint swelling and pain; muscle weakness and pain.
Skin, hair and nails	Cold extremities; athlete's foot; 'jock itch'; fungal toe and/or fingernails.
General	Feeling unwell and fatigued; frequent headaches or migraines; insomnia; craving sweet, starchy foods and alcohol; multiple chemical sensitivities; feeling worse in damp and mouldy places like cellars; feeling better on holiday/at the coast/in summer and worse in the autumn (fall).

presence of mercury which means that wherever mercury is stored, candidal overgrowth will be supported.

In nature, yeast spores which land on a fallen leaf, for instance, will change into their fungal form with mycelia that penetrate into the body of the leaf and that also perforate through the leaf where they release more spores. Normally our intestinal lining acts as a barrier between our tissues and the contents of our intestines which are technically outside the body and there is selective absorption of chemicals from digested food across this membrane. However, the 'roots' of the mycelial form of Candida penetrate between the cells of the intestinal lining and release spores – this time into the lymph and blood circulation of the host. By breaching this barrier the Candida is able to release the approximately 90 toxins that it produces into the body, making the host feel generally unwell. In the process, the Candida also creates a 'leaky gut', whereby foods are absorbed into the circulation before they are properly digested. These large food molecules are then identified by the immune system as 'foreign proteins' and attacked in the same way as a bacterial infection would be. In this fashion, multiple food intolerances can develop and become more severe and more numerous as the intestinal lining becomes ever more 'leaky'. In addition, the spores released into the circulation can colonize other organs by changing into their fungal forms and thus breaching their membranes. This process is responsible for the myriad different and often confusing symptoms of FRS detailed in figure 2.

Treatment of Candidiasis

Whilst treating candidal overgrowth with anti-fungal medications or herbs may provide some temporary relief from symptoms, some people can become indefinitely dependent upon these methods as they experience worse symptoms every time they try to wean themselves off the medications. Also, whilst the drugs kill Candida, they may allow other fungi and organisms to proliferate, thus compounding the problem. Candida is estimated to produce up to 400 highly toxic substances when it dies, and instigating a massive drug-induced Herxheimer reaction (die-off) in someone whose organs of excretion are already heavily compromised floods the system with toxins and can produce some very unpleasant symptoms. This approach most probably results in the re-storage of these toxins in possibly more vulnerable organs and tissues and this process is known as retoxification. Two of the drugs most commonly used (Ketaconozal and Nystatin) are quite toxic to the liver in addition to inducing die-off and may not cover the full spectrum of yeasts. The goal of effective treatment has to be to remove the cause – which is largely mercury – while supporting the organs of excretion and providing the high-quality nutrients the body requires to regenerate.

Viral Infections

Many viruses have the ability to lie low for decades and possibly lifetimes within the cells whilst evading destruction – and this is known as latency. This can be clearly witnessed in the particular case of an initial herpes simplex viral infection and the recurring cold sores that can affect the individual over a lifetime thereafter. As mercury

Figure 3: The main viruses associated with FRS

The herpes family of viruses	Illness and symptoms
Epstein-Barr virus (EBV) aka human herpes virus 4 (HHV4)	The most common virus in humans, carried by 90% of the population. Causes infectious mononucleosis or glandular fever, sometimes known as the 'kissing disease' because it can be transmitted in saliva. Symptoms include extreme tiredness, flu-like symptoms and a dry cough. Effects can be sudden and lasting as though 'someone put the lights out'. Blood tests can determine current or previous infection.
Cytomegalovirus (CMV) aka human herpes virus (HHV5)	From 'cyto' meaning cell and 'mega' meaning large. This is a virus to which we are nearly all exposed at some stage. It induces glandular fever-type symptoms and may specifically affect the salivary glands.
Varicella-zoster virus	The initial infection is chickenpox involving a blister-like rash on torso and face and is highly contagious. The virus can then lie dormant within the nerve roots and be reactivated, causing periodic subsequent bouts of shingles.
Human herpes virus 6 (HHV6)	Initial infection in childhood or adolescence/adulthood which may manifest as a glandular fever/mononucleosis-type illness that tests negative to CMV or EBV. Can become latent and reactivate when the immune system is compromised.
Herpes simplex viruses 1 & 2 (HSV1/HSV2)	Causes cold sores and genital herpes and can lie dormant in nerve roots with intermittent periods of reactivation. Very common.
Hepatitis B and Hepatitis C	Hepatitis B is contracted by contact with infected body fluids and Hepatitis C mostly by contact with infected blood, although sexual transmission is possible. Both specifically affect the liver producing pain over the right ribs, jaundice, possible foul-smelling breath, dark urine and pale stools. Blood tests will determine infection.
The enterovirus family	Illness and symptoms
Coxsackie virus	Produces mild flu-like symptoms and can affect the nervous system like its close relation, the polio virus. Implicated in Parkinsonism.
Hepatitis A	Affects the liver and is contracted from contaminated food.

toxicity is addressed, usually several latent viruses will appear that the body will require support in clearing. Although many viruses have been suspected of involvement in FRS including enterovirus, adenovirus, parvovirus and various so-called 'stealth' viruses, the spotlight seems to have fallen upon the herpes family of viruses. These viruses derive their name from the word 'to creep' and this refers to the insidious nature of their infection, latency and recurrence. Please see figure 3 for a list of these viruses and their associated illnesses.

Parasitic Infections

Unlike bacteria, fungi and viruses which may arise from within, parasites are acquired from the environment but find a supportive milieu in which to grow. A parasite is an organism that lives in or on a host and either feeds on the host's tissues or competes with the host for nutrients and usually produces substances that are toxic to the host. There are at least a hundred types of common human parasites ranging from the microscopic to large intestinal worms. Parasitic infections are actually very common, with only the obvious ones being acknowledged, such as head lice. In fact, they are the single biggest cause of death and illness in the world and half the population of the developed world carries at least one parasite – and a quarter of those have an active infection. Giardia lamblia is the fourth most common parasite in the world with one in five having been infected at some time in their lives; half of all sufferers of irritable bowel syndrome carry the parasite. Forty per cent of children in developed countries have had more than one parasitic infection and parasites are often a factor in chronic disease, with one in five chronically sick people testing positive for their presence. It is possible that the primary causes of parasitic infections include inadequate stomach acid (which kills parasite eggs) and inadequate digestive enzymes and bile. This means that improperly digested proteins can support parasite growth within the intestine.

Over the millennia, parasites have evolved sophisticated mechanisms to evade destruction by their host's immune system and to produce cravings for their preferred foodstuff in their host. They can also multiply at an incredible rate producing thousands of eggs a day and many parasites have developed a 'belt and braces' approach to avoiding removal such as the tapeworm, which attaches itself to the intestinal lining using both suckers and hooks. Many also have complex life cycles involving different hosts and quiescent and active phases, so laboratory tests often fail to correctly identify parasitic infections.

Sources of Parasites

Like fungal spores, parasite eggs are found everywhere. The most common method of transmission is through drinking contaminated water or eating undercooked meat or fish. Fruit and vegetables can be cross-contaminated during preparation by infected meat products or may carry soil that harbours eggs or cysts. Many cases of infection are through unwitting faecal–oral contact by those involved in food preparation or packing not washing their hands after going to the toilet. Other methods of transmission include direct sexual contact, inhaling contaminated dust, insect bites, walking barefoot and contact with infected pets or animals.

The Symptoms of Parasitic Infection

There is no part of the body that is immune to parasitic infection. One third of parasites inhabit the digestive tract, the other two-thirds invade the brain, the muscles, the heart, the thyroid gland and other tissues. The symptoms that parasites produce are many and varied and include: erratic bowel habits with alternating constipation and diarrhoea, foul-smelling stools, sore breasts (not related to the menstrual cycle), flu-like symptoms, an itchy anus (especially at night), weight loss and fatigue. Addressing an inadequate digestive system and the underlying metal toxicity will ultimately help the immune system to tackle these unwelcome guests.

Vaccinations

> The road to hell is paved with good intentions.
>
> **Samuel Johnson**

The term vaccination comes from the Latin 'vacca' for cow. Vaccination began in 1796 when Dr Edward Jenner injected pus from the blisters of a milkmaid suffering with cowpox into his gardener's young son. It had been observed that milkmaids who had contracted cowpox appeared immune to smallpox. This theory, happily, was borne out when he subsequently injected the child with smallpox and the boy did not contract the disease. Unfortunately, many of the viruses and other microbes that require treatment during a programme of metal detoxification appear to have been introduced, albeit unwittingly, by vaccinations. The technique for production of vaccines often involves taking pus or lymph from an infected person or animal and then cultivating it on decomposing animal tissue such as chicken eggs, monkey kidneys or aborted human foetuses. An adjuvant or poison such as aluminium sulphate is then added to this material in order to provoke an immune reaction when injected. This means that a two-month old baby in the US will have been exposed to more than 50 times the recommended 'safe' levels of aluminium by the vaccination schedule. This material is then preserved in a base containing such substances as mercury (thimerosal), formaldehyde or squalene. Vaccinations can introduce live material such as that used in the BCG, MMR, oral polio and chickenpox vaccines or 'inactivated' material such as that in the Polio (Salk), DPT, hepatitis B, HIB and meningitis vaccines.

A bit like a medieval castle, the body presents a series of defences that ramp up from being fairly general to highly specific as each layer is breached, with the production of antibodies by the immune system as the ultimate response. Initial defences include skin and mucous membranes and their secretions and the acid environment of the stomach which kills swallowed pathogens. The immune system functions by reacting to and 'memorizing' a particular protein on each pathogen. The researchers at the pharmaceutical companies try to establish which part of the microbe the immune system is responding to and then attempt to isolate and introduce this part in an inactivated form. The goal is to provoke the body into responding and storing the appropriate immune 'memory' without exposure to the dangerous pathogen.

Some problems inherent in this approach are listed below.

- The material may not be as harmless or as inactive as is assumed.
- We don't normally encounter three diseases at exactly the same time, however, with the DPT or MMR vaccines, several immune challenges are administered together. This may overwhelm the most robust of systems, but may prove especially challenging to the immature immune system of a young child.
- The effects of the toxic metals that are added to the vaccine are highly detrimental and synergistic. For example, the dose of aluminium and of mercury that would separately kill 1 per cent of laboratory rats, when combined kills *all* of the experimental rats.
- The chemical constituents such as thimerosal, aluminium sulphate and formaldehyde are injected along with possibly multiple pathogens and may combine to adversely affect the immune system.
- Many vaccinations are given long before the infant's immune system has had a chance to start functioning effectively and the sheer number of assaults on young immune systems may also be an issue. Children in the UK receive 9 vaccinations before the age of 3 years old and 16 vaccinations by 15 years of age and children in the US receive multiple vaccinations against 11 different diseases before the age of 6 years old.
- The exposure to multiple doses of the mercury preservative thimerosal alone may have very deleterious effects on the developing child.

- Normally when you encounter a pathogen, it has to breach all your outer defences before gaining entry to the inner sanctum of your circulation and immune system. When foreign substances are encountered in this way Th 1 lymphocytes are produced which results in lifelong immunity. With vaccination the infected material is introduced directly into the circulation without the priming that might have occurred if this were to happen naturally. Also, the immunity that vaccination provides may only be shortlived as it is Th 2 lymphocytes, rather than Th 1 lymphocytes, that are stimulated.
- The use of animal material in production means that the vaccine includes fragments of animal RNA and DNA. Other contaminants that have been identified include retro viruses (which can cause cancer in animals), simian (monkey) cytomegalovirus in polio vaccine and chicken viruses in measles vaccine.
- In addition to the additives mentioned elsewhere vaccines may also intentionally include phenol, acetone, glycerin and monosodium glutamate (MSG). Additionally and unintentionally they may also contain faecal matter, animal kidney or brain, animal blood and serum, yeast proteins and antibiotics.
- Perhaps most remarkably, *very few long-term studies have been done on the safety or efficacy of vaccinations*!
- Whilst vaccination may or may not afford protection from specific diseases, what price might we inadvertently be paying? Are the current explosions in the incidence of asthma, hyperactivity or autism a result? If vaccinations have life-long benefits as is claimed, why too can they not have life-long consequences?
- No meaningful data of adverse effects are kept as symptoms have to manifest within a remarkably short period of time to be legally attributed to the vaccine. However, the sudden illness of George Fisher, a healthy toddler, the day after vaccination and his subsequent death 10 days later was deemed by a UK court in 2008 to have occurred 'too soon' to have been caused by the vaccine!
- So keen are the medical profession on the vaccination programme, that they now want to introduce vaccinations for babies against hepatitis B and cervical cancer. The threat posed by these diseases may never be encountered and certainly not for decades, so is it entirely appropriate that young babies are subjected to this additional immune insult?
- Perhaps, most shockingly, there is *little evidence that vaccinations work*. Many people who have been vaccinated subsequently contract the disease that they

have been vaccinated against but doctors will attribute whooping cough to bronchitis or asthma for instance – assuming the vaccine to have been effective. Also, only 10 per cent of the world's population was ever vaccinated against smallpox and yet this disease died out in unvaccinated populations too.

- Vaccinosis is a term used by veterinarians to refer to the overuse of vaccinations producing chronic ill health and even death in animals, and you have to wonder why this is not also acknowledged in humans.
- There is a great deal of evidence to show that there had been a massive decline in incidence of many of the diseases that we vaccinate against *before* the vaccination programme was introduced. This can be attributed to the provision of clean water and proper sanitation, improved nutrition and hygiene, and better housing providing relief from the squalid and overcrowded conditions that the majority of people lived in.
- Fundamentally, these microbes may arise from *within* rather than infecting us from *without* as discussed previously, so the whole concept underlying vaccination may be based on a false premise.
- Last, but not least, the body does not need to be introduced to every pathogen it is ever likely to encounter in order to effectively combat it. The immune system works on the basis of defending against proteins it does not recognize (non-self) as opposed to those belonging to the body (self).

The harm for you may already have been done. However, where you can avoid the need for vaccination, such as choosing holidays that do not require vaccinations for tropical diseases like yellow fever, try to do so – at least until you are considerably stronger. If you have a child, make sure you *really understand the risks* you might be exposing your child to in having a vaccination. If there is any history of autism in your family, consider the consequences very carefully indeed, because an autistic spectrum response to vaccinations tends to run in families. Also, if your family has a history of immune disorders such as eczema, asthma or autoimmune disease, ensure that you are fully informed, as an adverse reaction to vaccination is more likely in these individuals.

Miasms

Before finally leaving the subject of infective organisms, it is worth mentioning the concept of miasms, created by the father of homeopathy Samuel Hahnemann in the 19th century. Miasms are predispositions to certain illnesses that have been handed down through generations from our antecedents who were exposed to the many plagues that swept through Europe in the Middle Ages. This has resulted in four pre-dispositions against which an individual may struggle for an entire lifetime unless treated. Most people carry two miasms (one from either parental line), and a practitioner versed in homeopathy will be able to address this aspect of treatment.

Dental Infections

The once widely accepted notion of 'foci of infection' fell out of favour in the 20th century, but is being embraced again in the light of recent evidence. The concept is that the mouth in particular can become a reservoir from which infective agents can colonize other regions in the body and from which their noxious products can spread, affecting overall health. The three main oral sources of infection that the FRS sufferer needs to be aware of are addressed below.

Root-Filled Teeth

The body of the tooth is composed of dentine (ivory) which is formed from hundreds of thousands of tiny tubules that run from its surface to the central chamber within that contains the nerves and blood and lymph vessels (the pulp). In a single-rooted incisor (front tooth) there is an estimated 5 km (3 miles) of tubing and in a molar (back tooth) there may be as much as 12 km (10 miles). In addition, the pulp canals within the tooth (normally one per root) have many tiny lateral canals that provide accessory circulation and perforate the body of the tooth from the surface to the interior. Endodontically treated ('endo-' means within and '-dont' means tooth) or root-filled teeth in which the dead or dying pulp has been removed and the canals have been cleaned and filled have, by definition, no circulation. It is claimed that the normally benign streptococcal bacteria – especially the diplococci and short-chain Streptococcus viridans – mutate into their pathogenic forms in the absence of oxygen. This occurs in the 30 per cent of teeth with additional canals which may have been missed, in the tiny lateral canals and in the vast system of dentinal tubules. These bacteria can then release very toxic substances that cannot be combated by the immune system. Some teeth present an obvious problem on x-ray, with a dark shadow of a cavity produced by fibrous or abscessed tissue showing clearly against the lighter surrounding bone. However, many x-rays miss infections that lie in front of or behind the tooth being x-rayed. Any tooth with a poor root-filling or such an area is suspect, as is any tooth that you know to occasionally get infected or to be problematic.

The early 20th-century dentist and nutritionist, Dr Weston Price, found pus to be sterile and an indicator of successful quarantine by the body. What is claimed, however, is that in those with severely compromised immune systems, the body is unable to mount a response to this toxic assault and so there are *no overt signs* of a problem on an x-ray. For this reason, some authorities recommend the removal of *all* root-filled teeth if you are seriously or chronically ill. Consulting a kinesiologist or a practitioner skilled in Vega testing or using the DIY muscle testing outlined in the Appendix may indicate whether a tooth is likely to be a problem. Alternatively, you will have to make this decision for yourself, taking into consideration the chronology of your illness and how it relates to any dental treatment or problems and, ultimately, how compromised your health is. Dr Price considered that if the previous two generations of your family have been resistant to degenerative diseases, then root-fillings are not normally likely to present an issue. However, he found that those with a family history of serious illness were more vulnerable to the adverse effects of root-fillings. Certainly some root-fillings (historically probably the majority in the UK) have been done using a filling material which combines an antibiotic and a steroid paste rather than compacting a relatively inert material to obturate the canal system of the tooth. These teeth can certainly present a toxic cocktail when opened, frequently smelling awful. Another sign that many dentists might pass over as being of no consequence is that of condensing osteitis (oss-tee-i-tis), which shows as a dense white area around the tip of the root, and this can also indicate a toxicity problem originating from the tooth.

'Cavitations'

Also implicated are neuralgia-inducing cavitational osteonecrotic (NICO) lesions or what have come to be known as 'cavitations' which occur when a tooth – possibly infected – was extracted without removal of the surrounding periodontal membrane (the fibrous 'joint' that attaches teeth to the jawbone). These can subsequently form 'chambers' within the bone which can harbour anaerobic bacteria which produce toxins such as hydrogen sulphide and methylthiol which can then enter the circulation, detrimentally affecting the body. Cavitations most commonly appear at the sites of lower molar and lower wisdom tooth extraction.

Gum Disease

The majority of people also have some degree or other of periodontal disease (also known as periodontitis or gum disease) and this, too, can be the site of a large number of anaerobic bacteria gaining ready access to the body. It is estimated that the infected area (although hidden from view) is equivalent to that of a tennis ball in someone with moderate periodontal disease. Healthy gums do not bleed, so if you think you may have gum disease and don't feel that your dentist is addressing the problem properly, ask for a referral to a periodontist (gum specialist). This may cost some serious money for deep cleaning around the roots of all your teeth and you will have to be diligent yourself about brushing and flossing on a daily basis thereafter.

It certainly seems to be worth asking your dentist if any of your teeth seem chronically infected or if there are any apparent cavitations on x-ray. If you have a troublesome tooth or teeth that you have been 'hanging on to' and you have an FRS it would seem to be a good idea to consider the possibility of extracting the affected teeth. It is also worth taking good daily care of your mouth by brushing with a non-fluoride toothpaste and flossing as well as seeing the hygienist and/or dentist regularly. Dental treatment is discussed further in chapter 18.

Chapter 9
Toxic Metals

Metals

There are just over a hundred known elements, and of those, nearly three-quarters are metals. These metals share certain physical characteristics; one of their distinguishing features is their willingness to donate electrons, which means that they can become positively charged ions and conduct heat and electricity. Metals will readily lose these electrons (even just in moist air) and the metal ions that result are then water-soluble. Some elements exhibit characteristics of both metals and non-metals and are known as metalloids or semi-metals, an example of which is arsenic. The metals silver and gold belong to the same group in the periodic table as copper, for instance, and so share many properties; as do cadmium and mercury which are in the same group as zinc.

Minerals

Metal ions which occur naturally in biologically available forms in combination with substances such as carbonate or phosphate are known as minerals and are essential for many physiological processes. These minerals serve many important functions in the body, for example, calcium gives structure to bone. In addition, all proteins are chains of amino acids that are folded into complex three-dimensional shapes that are critical to their recognition and function in the body and it is often a metal ion that is involved in this process. The iron in haemoglobin, for instance, is integral to both its oxygen-carrying capacity and the shape of the molecule, and magnesium is critical to the elaborate structure of DNA. Other minerals, such as biologically-available selenium, act as antioxidants and help prevent cancer, and many minerals serve as the cofactors which are essential to many biochemical reactions in the body. Some metals, however, have no known function and there is believed to be no safe lower limit of exposure to these metals, for which reason they are known as toxic metals.

Toxic Metals

It is only with the heart that one can see rightly; what is essential is invisible to the eye.

Antoine de Saint-Exupéry

A quarter of the Earth's mass is comprised of metals, although there is a smaller percentage at the crust. Man has mined and refined these surface metals and uses them in seemingly innocuous everyday items such as aluminium foil packaging, mercury in vaccinations, copper water piping and nickel in hydrogenated fats. Some people are also occupationally exposed to the metals used in manufacturing, scientific or laboratory settings and some through hobbies such as making stained-glass windows (lead) or developing photographs (silver).

Whilst some minerals are essential to the function of the body, metals in their refined form are of no use and are often toxic. All metals have the potential to be toxic, depending upon the dose and even in biologically available forms the difference between a therapeutic amount of a mineral and a toxic dose can be very small. The human body has developed sophisticated mechanisms for transporting and storing essential minerals and also for eliminating toxic or non-essential metals such as the synthesis of metallothioneins primarily in the liver and kidneys.

The term 'toxic metal' is used to refer to metals that have no known biological function and disrupt essential physiological processes and includes such metals as mercury, lead, aluminium, cadmium, barium and uranium. Other metals can become toxic in specific forms, for example, chromium as the Cr^{3+} ion is essential for maintaining blood sugar levels, but in the Cr^{6+} form is a carcinogen. The term 'heavy metal' is falling out of favour as it has no generally accepted meaning, however it is often used to refer to toxic metals of high atomic weight, such as cadmium, lead and mercury. There are exceptions, however, such as molybdenum, which is an essential heavy metal and beryllium which is a light, but very toxic metal. In 1974, the World Health Organization acknowledged that heavy metal toxicity was a *major cause* of world disease.

Allopathic medicine classifies toxic metal exposure as either being acute (two weeks or less), intermediate (between two weeks and a year) or chronic (more than one year). Unfortunately, we know what we do about metal poisoning because of some infamous incidents of accidental exposure or through chronic exposure of the workforce in industries where toxic metals have been used. For instance, the use of lead cups by the ruling classes of the Roman Empire often resulted in madness and sterility and is thought to have contributed to the fall of the Empire. Physicians, too, have played their part in administering these toxic materials 'therapeutically' over the millennia. What we are concerned with, however, is chronic, low-level exposure over a period of decades whereby the elimination channels are overwhelmed and the toxic metal accumulates in the body.

What Makes Toxic Metals Toxic?

Toxic metals can disrupt many body processes and their effects can be insidious and hard to detect. Metal toxicity also has symptoms that are easily mistaken for a host of other, commonly occurring conditions such as rheumatoid arthritis and autoimmune diseases (and is probably the unseen cause). Toxic metals can interfere with normal biological function in a number of ways:

- Heavy metals attach to the sulphhydryl group (–SH or thiol group) in biological proteins, disrupting function and forming very secure complexes that are extremely hard to dislodge. This process leads to the bioaccumulation of heavy metals up the food chain and is the reason why we need to limit our consumption of the bigger carnivorous fish. The heavy metals also inactivate enzymes and disrupt cell membrane function, cause cross-linking of proteins and generally reduce the detoxification capacity and the biochemical function of the individual.
- Toxic metals also attach to mineral binding sites either through deficiency of the required mineral or an excess of the toxic metal. The endocrine glands, for example, all have a high requirement for minerals such as selenium and zinc and these mineral binding sites can be rendered ineffective by binding heavy or toxic metals such as mercury.
- Toxic metals can bind firmly to the oxygen-transporting binding sites in the haemoglobin of red blood cells and are believed to do so for the life of the cell. This means that the oxygen-carrying capacity of the blood is severely reduced, profoundly affecting all organs and systems, although red blood cell counts may be normal.
- The thyroid hormone thyroxine contains four iodine molecules which, if one or more are replaced by a toxic metal, will render the hormone ineffective although, again, blood tests will reveal circulating thyroxine levels to be within normal limits.
- Toxic metals can substitute for the essential metal ions in proteins, thus altering the shape of the protein and rendering it functionless, or if the protein is an enzyme, rendering it ineffective. Sometimes the body 'mistakes' a toxic metal for an essential mineral with similar properties, such as cadmium which can replace the zinc in proteins that is essential to their structure or

function. In this way lead is thought to substitute for structural calcium in bone to manifest as osteoporosis.

- Toxic metals may also bind to the cell receptors intended for docking substances such as insulin or thyroxine with the effect that circulating amounts are normal but the cells are functionally deficient.
- Metal ions can also either remove or donate electrons to other molecules and this can result in disruption of function, premature ageing and the mutations that can cause cancer if the DNA bases are affected.

These are all subtle and cumulative changes that are hard to detect but can have a devastating effect on the body over a period of decades, often ultimately resulting in death. Occult metal toxicity may play a causative role in *nearly all serious and chronic illness* and is certainly the primary cause of fatigue-related syndromes.

Some other factors that may also enhance metal toxicity include:

- A relative deficiency of the essential minerals derived from whole foods, vegetables, nuts and seeds.
- Synergistic interactions between metals which greatly magnify the toxic potential of the metals involved.
- Some metals such as lead are mobilized depending upon the phosphate/calcium balance of the diet.
- Some substances may enhance absorption of toxic metals, for instance, coffee is thought to escort aluminium into the brain.
- Various forms of electromagnetic radiation are also believed to promote metal toxicity.

Signs of Metal Toxicity

Please refer to figure 4 for some of the tests that can be performed to assess metal toxicity. Please note that whilst mercury toxicity may not show in hair analysis, urine, stool or blood samples, this does *not rule out the possibility of mercury toxicity* in the brain and other body compartments. Note that fractionated urinary porphyrins can be used as an indirect measure of the presence of heavy metals, since porphyrins are involved in the haemoglobin pathway which becomes deranged as a result of their presence. The development of white bands or patches on the finger- and toenails known as Mees' lines can also indicate recent exposure to, or mobilization of, heavy metals. These tests may or may not aid your understanding of your condition for a variety of reasons. However, if you have a history of occupational exposure to any metals or have (or had) dental amalgam fillings or vaccinations and if you suffer from any of the following, the chances are high that you have significant metal toxicity:

Figure 4: Tests for toxic metals

Pros	Cons
Hair analysis	
This is relatively inexpensive, but will only reveal toxic metals in circulation recently. Available at: www.genovadiagnostics.com	Does not show historic exposure to metals or those stored in body compartments. When conducted on autistic children, toxic metals were notably absent, leading to the conclusion that those who are unable to excrete toxic metals are the most vulnerable to bioaccumulation and that this test only indicates which metals the body is able to *excrete*. Using hair colourants may affect this test.
Home urine/saliva tests	
These are inexpensive and can be obtained for home use over the Internet. A variety of tests are available that assess aspects of general heavy metal toxicity and specific metals. Check: www.genovadiagnostics.com	Will not show metals in storage, but may give a good indication of issues.
Kelmer test	
In this test, urine samples are tested before and after a chelating agent such as DMSA (a binding agent) is given to provoke the release of toxic metals from storage in body compartments. Can perform home test as above.	Adverse reactions are possible, as routes of excretion may be overwhelmed by the quantity of toxic metals mobilized from storage. Some suggest a small provocation test to determine if metal toxicity is an issue. If attending laboratory/clinic – time and expense.
Memory lymphocyte immuno stimulation assay (MELISA)	
A blood sample is sent for assessment of type IV allergic reactions to metals. Contact: www.melisa.org	Assesses allergy, not toxicity.
Fat biopsy	
Here, a small amount of fat is analysed for toxins.	Invasive and unpleasant, expensive, requires doctor/surgeon.

- Any fatigue-related syndrome and/or any serious, degenerative, chronic or autoimmune disease.
- *Any* condition that is failing to respond to treatment or that is getting worse instead of better.
- *Any* 'mystery' or 'invisible' illness that the doctors cannot identify and where test results come back 'normal'.
- Chronic or recurrent candidal infections and/or any frequent or chronic infections.
- Any contact sensitivity to metals.

Figure 4: cont.

Pros	Cons
Whole blood/serum tests	
Blood/serum analysed for circulating toxins. Available at: www.genovadiagnostics.com	A clinician is required to take the blood sample. Will not show metals in storage in body compartments. The body will prioritize storage of the most damaging substances from circulation so that blood tests are only of limited value.
Sweat test	
With this test, a patch is stuck on the skin for a period of a couple of hours and then the sweat collected is analysed.	Have to go to laboratory and wait for 2 or more hours. It is possible if you also have hypothyroidism that you may sweat less than others, invalidating the comparison.
Muscle testing	
This technique applies gentle pressure to a muscle in order to determine whether a substance stresses or supports the body. This binary system of muscles locking and unlocking can be used to communicate with the bio-computer in the brain and is the basis of kinesiology. Non-invasive, gentle (ideally!) and relatively inexpensive. No test is infallible, but a good kinesiologist should get close. Can reveal stored toxins.	Routine muscle testing may not indicate metal toxicity (or the extent of metal toxicity) unless particular techniques have been used to reveal their presence to the bio-computer (brain) first. This is because the metals were absorbed into the autonomic nervous system under the control of the emotional right brain and the bio-computer is unaware of their presence.
Vega testing	
Test substances are introduced into the Vega machine and the response of the energy circuits of the body assessed. Non-invasive, relatively cheap, widely available and may indicate the presence of stored metals.	Reliability may depend upon practitioner.

Some sufferers and their practitioners are very committed to identifying a specific causative toxic metal or metals before initiating treatment. However, this is not strictly necessary because the treatment suggested in this book will work for most metal toxicities. Some also prefer to obtain proof positive of allergic reactions to toxic metals such as mercury before proceeding with treatment, but I wonder if they would apply this same logic if it were arsenic toxicity at issue? The proof of the diagnosis will be in the treatment and the permanence of the solution.

Sources of Metals

Many metals may be involved in FRS depending upon a history of exposure and the individual's emotional and biochemical vulnerability at the time. Please examine

Figure 5: The sources and symptoms of metal toxicity

Sources	Symptoms

Aluminium

Foodstuffs: Additives; cheese products; baking powder; white flour products; juice/milk in Tetrapaks; canned drinks and foods; beer from casks; foods packed in aluminium foil; foods cooked in aluminium cookware; table salt; tea bags. Tap water is often treated with aluminium sulphate and/or aluminium fluoride. NB: Aluminium competes with magnesium for absorption in the intestine and non-dairy creamer, citric acid and calcium citrate supplements can all enhance aluminium absorption, as can calcium deficiency.
Pharmaceuticals: Antacids; buffered aspirin; nasal sprays; over-the-counter painkillers; douches.
Personal care: Astringents; antiperspirants; lipstick and other cosmetics; toothpaste; hair spray.
Other: Naturally occurring in air, soil and water; exhaust fumes; tobacco smoke and fireworks.

Physical: Believed to accumulate in the brain possibly causing Alzheimer's disease and motor neuron disease; lung damage; loss of coordination; balance problems; osteoporosis; kidney problems; impaired liver function; digestive problems – particularly affecting the gall bladder and causing referred pain to the shoulder; anaemia; rickets; aching muscles; seizures; dizziness; tiredness; headaches and speech problems.
Psychological: Confusion; dementia; memory loss; reduced mental alertness; extreme nervousness; hyperactivity and learning disorders in children.

Arsenic – No 1 ATSDR list*

Foodstuffs: Contamination of ground/well water, wine and herbal preparations possible.
Household: Ceramics; copper; glass; wallpaper; weedkiller; insecticide.
Other: Industrial exposure.

Physical: Poisons energy production in all organ systems; numbness, tingling or burning of the hands and/or feet; restless and fidgety; drowsiness; an agonized expression; short menstrual cycle; dermatitis; headaches; fatigue; kidney and liver damage; hair loss; muscle weakness; periods of being unable to stand; sleeping with arms raised; food allergies and seizures. A carcinogen – especially lung and skin.
Psychological: Anguish; fear of death and being alone; fearful dreams; fear and worry; selfishness; may self-harm; suicidal.

Cadmium – No 7 ATSDR list*

Foodstuffs: Coffee; fish and shellfish; organ meat; dairy products and soft tap water.
Household: Some red and yellow paints; coloured plastics (including dentures); ceramics; fertilizer; fungicide; pesticide; antiseptic; leather; some batteries.
Industrial: Ore smelting and processing; electroplating; welding; burning of fossil fuels; spraying/removing paints; municipal waste.
Other: Biggest source for many is cigarette and tobacco smoke; exhaust fumes.

Physical: Foetal growth retardation; nausea; respiratory problems; sore joints; scaly skin; hair loss; weight loss; anaemia; kidney and liver damage; calcium stone formation; low blood haemoglobin levels; benign swelling of the prostate gland; fatigue; headaches; high blood pressure; osteoporosis; and an impaired immune system causing secondary infections and cancer.
Psychological: Irritability; learning disabilities; dementia.

Copper

Foodstuffs: Some meat.
Pharmaceutical: Intrauterine devices; contraceptive pill and some prescription medicines.
Household: Cookware; copper piping and water heating cylinders; fungicide.
Other: Air-conditioning systems and smoking.

Physical: Headaches; low blood sugar; poor digestion; increased heart rate; nausea; brain damage; liver damage; kidney damage; anaemia; deterioration of eyesight; hair loss in women; fatigue; skin rashes and premenstrual syndrome.
Psychological: 'Spaciness'; detachment; learning disorders; paranoia; depression; insomnia; psychosis and schizophrenia-type symptoms.
In children: Hyperactivity; ADD; ear infections; dyslexia and autism-type symptoms.

Figure 5: cont.

Sources	Symptoms
Gold **Pharmaceutical:** Drugs for rheumatoid arthritis and some skin diseases. **Other:** Electroplating; jewellery; gold crowns and bridges.	**Physical:** Dermatitis; hypersensitivity; seizures; kidney and/or liver damage. **Psychological:** Confusion.
Lead – No 2 ATSDR list* **Foodstuffs:** Water supplies from lead plumbing. **Household:** Paint chips and dust; lead-based paints; newsprint; insecticides; varnishes; certain plastics; heavy greases; leaded china. **Personal care:** Some lipsticks – especially long-lasting. **Industrial:** Solder; dyes; plumbing; pigments; enamels and glazes. **Other:** Soil and air in industrial areas; leaded petrol.	**Physical:** Dyslexia; epilepsy; fatigue; poor coordination; weight loss; gout; pallor; glaucoma; paralysis; insomnia; tremors; metallic taste; a blue line along the gums; dropping of the ankles or wrists; osteomalacia and rickets; anaemia; blindness; colic; abdominal cramping and excessive intestinal gas; constipation; immunosuppression; infertility; liver dysfunction; hypertension; kidney dysfunction; weakness; wasting of shoulder muscles; chest pain; feeling worse at night; seizures; coma and death. May be involved in multiple sclerosis. Exposure as a child strongly associated with increased mortality. **Psychological:** Hallucinations; hyperactivity; irritability; memory loss; nightmares; impaired learning; and schizophrenia. Implicated in impulsivity and violent crime.
Manganese **Industrial:** Affects mainly men through occupational exposure as welders, railroad workers, miners, steel workers and through exposure to fertilizers. **Other:** Also found in contaminated air, water and soil in industrial areas.	**Physical:** Manganism or 'Welder's disease' may be mistaken for Parkinson's disease. Includes generalized muscle weakness; slurred speech; poor balance and co-ordination; respiratory difficulties; kidney and/or liver damage; difficulty with facial expression; reduced white blood cell counts; sexual dysfunction; impotence and foetal damage in pregnant women. **Psychological:** 'Manganese madness', i.e.: antisocial behaviour involving minor compulsive acts, emotional instability and hallucinations. Implicated in violent crime.
Nickel **Foodstuffs:** Peanut butter; hydrogenated oils; tea/coffee machines. Also naturally high in chocolate, soy products, nuts and oatmeal. **Other:** Jewellery; prosthetics; smoking; contaminated soil, air or water.	**Physical:** Haemorrhages; low blood pressure; nausea, skin problems and fibromyalgia.
Platinum Jewellery and used in cancer treatment.	Urticaria or dermatitis and respiratory disorders including sneezing, shortness of breath or asthma.
Silver Jewellery, wound dressings and medicines.	Heart and liver disorders.

*Agency for Toxic Substance and Disease Registry, United States Department of Health and Human Services

figure 5 which outlines several of the main metals implicated in FRS and consider whether any of the symptom pictures are familiar and whether you may have had any exposure – witting or unwitting – to this metal. A significant toxin burden may have come from your mother so examine her history of exposure, health and dental history in this new light. If you think that one or more of these metals may be playing a role in your FRS you may wish to be tested to this metal to satisfy your own curiosity, but it will not really alter treatment. The mother of all toxic metals, however, is mercury and it is to this beautiful and deadly metal that we now turn our attention.

Mercury Toxicity

> Mercury is the hottest, the coldest, a true healer, a wicked murderer, a precious medicine, and a deadly poison, a friend that can flatter and lie.
>
> **J Woodall, 1639**

Mercury is the most harmful naturally occurring substance and rates as the third most toxic substance known on the Agency for Toxic Substance and Disease Registry in the US. The Toxicity Centre at the University of Tennessee also rates poisons for their lethal toxicity to humans and grades the most deadly – plutonium – at 1,900 and mercury at 1,600. Mercury is a very potent neurotoxin (attracted to nervous tissue) and is a far more powerful biological toxin than either lead or arsenic. The World Health Organization has determined that there is *no safe lower dose* and even one molecule of mercury will cause some tissue damage. Mercury can also produce and perpetuate symptoms in any organ system and amplify the effects of all other toxins.

A History of Mercury Poisoning

Man has a long and troubled history of fascination with mercury and its properties. The first Emperor of China was ironically killed by the mercury pills he was taking for immortality. The composer Amadeus Mozart and many of his contemporaries in Vienna died of the mercury they were taking as a cure for syphilis. When it comes to environmental mercury exposure, two of the most infamous examples took place in Japan in the early part of the 20th century. The Chisso Corporation polluted the waters of Minimata with waste mercury and this bio-accumulated in the fish supplies killing many thousands of people and probably affecting hundreds of thousands more. Sadly, because of the politicking and denials of the cause a similar incident was later to occur at Niigata, Japan causing more human devastation. In another incident in the 1970s, grain that had been treated with a mercury fungicide and that was intended for planting was ordered by Saddam Hussein's regime in Iraq and supplied mostly to the Kurds in the north of the country. The desperate peasants ate rather than planted this grain and this led to an estimated 6,000 deaths and 100,000 people injured. In living memory mercury has been used in medications and pharmaceuticals. In the 1950s it was finally recognized that acrodynia or pink disease was caused by the use of mercuric compounds in Calomel powder which was used for teething in babies and the product was withdrawn.

Environmental Sources of Mercury

Whilst volcanoes are a natural source of atmospheric mercury, two-thirds of the remaining environmental mercury is thought to originate from coal-fired power stations, such as those currently being built in China. Mercury has been extensively used in industry in the production of gold, tin, cement, steel, batteries and explosives and is also widely used in laboratories and hospitals. The waste products from these plants are regarded as an 'external cost' and one for which companies are currently not held liable. This mercury contaminates the soil, water and air and is converted to organic mercury primarily by microbes. It then bio-accumulates and bio-concentrates up the food chain until finally being consumed by humans. Sadly, even crematoria release significant mercury vapours as the cadavers are cremated, although some countries are now introducing a requirement that they filter their emissions. Dental surgery wastes too are estimated to be responsible for one-third of the mercury in the sewage system and whilst some conscientious dentists fit separators there is, as yet, no requirement to do so in most countries.

Occupational Exposure to Mercury

It is recognized by the World Health Organization and various other health and safety organizations that those in some occupations are particularly at risk from mercury toxicity and there are strict occupational exposure limits. Historically, the Spanish Conquistadors mined mercury in Peru, using indigenous Indians as forced labour. Although they were only required to work six months once every two years, none of the miners were recorded to have survived this regime for more than four years. More recently, mercury was used to treat pelts in the hatting industry and this caused neurological problems including madness, which was probably the inspiration for Lewis Carroll's Mad Hatter character in *Alice in Wonderland*.

One of the groups with the greatest occupational exposure is dentists and their chairside assistants. At autopsy, the pituitary glands of dentists have been found to contain

800 times and the thyroid gland to contain *10 times* the mercury of the general population (who also probably have elevated levels). Many studies have shown that dentists have significantly compromised cognitive and behavioural skills compared to control groups. Dentists are also known to have one of the highest chemical and alcohol dependency and marital breakdown rates and up to seven times the suicide rate of other professions. One study found dentists to have an average of four times the mercury in their urine and another found seven times the mercury in their kidneys at autopsy compared to non-dental personnel and so it may not be surprising that dentists suffer significantly more kidney disorders than the rest of the population. The levels of mercury in hair and nail samples from dentists were up to three times those found in the general population with female personnel exhibiting higher levels than their male counterparts. A not unrelated fact may be that female dental workers are *three and a half times* more likely to suffer sterility, miscarriage and still birth. All chair-side dental personnel also have a higher incidence of brain, heart and lung cancers and other lung disorders.

> **Very few mercury exposed workers reached old age, and it was said that even if they did not die young, their health was so terribly undermined that they prayed for death.**
>
> **Dr Bernardino Ramazzini, the founder of occupational medicine**

Non-Occupational Exposure to Mercury

Most people will have some exposure to mercury from fish sources (see chapter 14) and from the mercury preservative thimerosal, used in many vaccinations. Other sources include: paint, tattoos, fabric softener, adhesives, ointments, antiseptics, floor wax, energy saving and fluorescent light bulbs, and cosmetics (look for 'mer' anywhere in the list of contents, e.g. thi*mer*osal). However, the World Health Organization conceded in 1991 that dental amalgam fillings represent the biggest source of mercury exposure for most people (65–90 per cent of body burden). The average amalgam filling contains approximately 1 gram of mercury and so the average adult is exposed to the timed release of a total of approximately 5 grams of mercury from their amalgam fillings over time. According to a 1991 study by Dr Chew(!) at the National University of Singapore, this average amalgam filling releases about 34mcg of mercury per day compared to a total of 2.3mcg exposure from fish and seafood sources. Direct correlations have been established between the number of amalgam fillings and the amount of mercury in the body. In the massive US Center for Disease Control National Health and Nutrition Examination Survey of the general population in 2001 the number of amalgam fillings was *significantly correlated* to the incidence of *many serious and degenerative disorders* including *cancer and multiple sclerosis.* The US Center for Disease Control also estimates that up to 8 per cent of the population have blood levels that exceed guideline 'safe' amounts.

Dental Amalgam

> Mercury amalgams are as close as you can get to the centre of the illness universe; their use in dentistry has set us up for most of the health problems we see today.
>
> **Dr Bruce Shelton MD, MD(H), DiHom, FBIH**

Dental amalgam accounts for about 80 per cent of all fillings placed and has been extensively used in dentistry for 190 years because it is cheap, easy to use, durable and hitherto regarded as safe. It is an approximately 50:50 mix of liquid mercury and silver alloy powder containing small quantities of other metals such as copper, zinc, nickel and tin. There are strict rules governing the storage of the material before placement of a filling and relating to the disposal of the 'toxic waste' produced and any accidental spills. All of which makes you wonder why the authorities think that the mouth of a human being would be a safe place to store this toxic substance in the interim! The official line maintained by the American Dental Association and other bodies for several decades now is that 'When mercury is combined with the metal used in dental amalgam, its toxic properties are made harmless' (ADA 1984). The authorities concede, however, that amalgam fillings emit a small but continuous amount of mercury vapour throughout their lifetime. In fact, it is now known that within seven years of placement, amalgam fillings have released *over half* their mercury content into their unfortunate owner's body and this figure rises to 80 per cent after 20 years. Some claim that dental amalgam never truly sets, but that it forms different microscopic alloy 'cells', effectively becoming a very stiff liquid. This may be evidenced by one of the problems with amalgam fillings known as 'creep'. This refers to the fact that amalgam swells over the cavity borders with time and little bits 'chip off', producing ditching and potential leakage.

A Brief History of Dental Amalgam

Dental amalgam was first introduced to the US in the early part of the 19th century by two of the five dentist Crawcour brothers from London, who promoted it under the grand title of Royal Mineral Succedaneum. There ensued the first 'amalgam war' as these brothers took patients from local dentists and this caused such a furore that just two years after the formation of the American Society of Dental Surgeons they decreed that the use of amalgam represented malpractice. The argument ignited again in 1920 and is known as the second amalgam war. The most recent 'third amalgam war' was started essentially by the US anti-amalgam dentist Dr Hal Huggins in 1973 and rages to this day. In response to the controversy, the American Dental Association decreed in 1986 that the removal of dental amalgam in the non-allergic patient was 'improper and unethical' and has maintained that stance ever since.

Muddy Waters

All five elements found in amalgam are known to adversely affect all the major organ systems and whilst the full effects of combining mercury with the other metals in dental amalgam are not fully understood, zinc alone is known to increase the toxicity of mercury many fold. Radioactive thallium is often a contaminant of mercury and may also be present in small amounts. The adverse effects of this are rarely immediately obvious and there are other factors which determine how much mercury leaches out, where it deposits and how it manifests. There is often, too, an extended latency period between exposure and the appearance of symptoms which means that researchers and sufferers do not make the causal link. This may be because the extensive intercellular matrix around the cells is used for storage before the mercury finally penetrates the inner confines of the cells, producing symptoms. Mercury is also known to track up the autonomic nerves that supply the various organs and this too will cause a delay between exposure and the gradual onset of symptoms. There is also a huge individual variability in the capacity to detoxify mercury, nutritional status and requirements and all of these factors conspire to confound and confuse researchers.

The Mouth Electric

The mechanism behind release of mercury vapour from dental amalgam is believed to be that once the components are mixed and inserted, galvanic currents occur between the different microscopic alloy phases that form within the body of the filling. Each filling also becomes electrically active within the wider environment of the mouth and the other 17 metals that may be present in crowns, bridges, posts, orthodontic braces and dentures, with saliva acting as a conductor. This is similar to the way Alessandro Volta created the first battery in 1800 by combining dissimilar metals with salt water. This process results in the most electrically active fillings giving off the most mercury vapour and may account for the metallic taste experienced by many individuals. This is graphically demonstrated in the 'smoking tooth' video (available on YouTube and at www.thenaturalrecoveryplan.com) which shows plumes of mercury vapour being given off an old amalgam filling in an extracted tooth illuminated against a phosphorescent screen. Patients with autoimmune diseases, multiple sclerosis, epilepsy and depression are often found to have a lot of high-negative-current fillings. Galvanic currents also result in crevice corrosion and the production of up to 16 different corrosion products (according to the late UK anti-amalgam activist Dr Jack Levenson) which are then abraded by eating or tooth-brushing, or chip off and are swallowed.

Another form of galvanic current is that established between the mucous membrane (which serves as a cathode) and the amalgam (which acts as an anode). This is thought to be the unseen mechanism that drives mercury into the tissues and jawbone. It has been demonstrated that tissue mercury levels in those with gold crowns or bridges placed on top of amalgam bases (known as 'cores') can reach over 20 times those of amalgam-free controls and is even higher in the bone surrounding the root tips of these teeth. This mechanism is also probably responsible for producing so-called amalgam 'tattoos', where the gums, lips or cheeks can become stained black. When removing old amalgam fillings I had always assumed the discolouration of the tooth to be due to corrosive products. I now know that these were scorch marks left by the electrical activity of the filling.

Figure 6: Relationships of teeth to meridians and organs

Teeth	Meridians	Location of symptoms (on same side)
Incisors	Kidney and bladder	Back of knee and ankle; hip; tonsils; sinuses; ovary; uterus; prostate; testicles and rectum.
Canines (cuspid)	Liver and gall bladder	Back of knee; hip; outside ankle; minor sinuses, tonsils; eye; hypothalamus. Lower canines only: ovaries/testes.
Premolars (bicuspids)	Spleen and stomach	Front of hip/knee; inside ankle; sinus; throat; thyroid; parathyroid gland. Upper jaw: breast and TMJ. Lower jaw: shoulder.
First and second molars	Lung and large intestine	Arms; feet; minor sinuses; bronchi; nose; breast. Upper jaw: shoulder. Lower jaw: TMJ, ovaries and testes.
Third molar (wisdom teeth)	Heart, small intestine, circulation sex (sex hormones) and triple warmer (mostly thyroid function)	Shoulder; arms; hands; sacroiliac region; foot; middle ear; CNS; anterior pituitary.

As advised by Dr Dietrich Klinghardt

A separate but related concern is that these fillings are producing currents and electrical potentials that are much greater than those employed by the nervous system. Whilst the brain operates at just a few millivolts, spikes of activity measuring *one thousand times* that figure – one volt – have been recorded from dental restorations. It is thought that this electrical activity might interfere with normal nerve transmission or functioning of the adjacent brain producing headaches, migraines, dizziness and nausea. The cells are known to act as capacitors which are organized and orientated electromagnetically and also to maintain a specific electrical potential across the cell membrane and it is not understood what effect these galvanic currents may have upon these delicate mechanisms. In Traditional Chinese Medicine, the teeth have energy meridians which run through them serving the vital organs, and the placing of any metal, especially an electromagnetically active one, may interfere with these energy flows. Figure 6 shows the organ systems believed to be related to the various teeth and you may be able to relate symptoms to a particular tooth in this way.

High-Copper Amalgam

So-called high-copper amalgam (or non-gamma II amalgam) was introduced in the mid-1970s to combat the problem of corrosion which was thought to lead to a lot of cracked and fractured teeth. This formulation contains approximately 30 per cent copper and in addition to releasing copper vapour, it has been demonstrated to form droplets of liquid mercury on the surface of the fillings and so release *50 times* the mercury vapour of the previous formulation. This one fact alone could lead to an epidemic of fatigue-related syndromes and other serious disorders and may account for the general rise in doctor's consultations and the precipitous decline in both male and female fertility recently.

Contributory Factors

To complicate matters further, electromagnetic fields are also thought to induce a current in dental amalgam fillings and increase the effects of galvanism. Both chewing (especially gum) and consuming hot and acidic foods and drinks have been shown to temporarily increase the release of mercury vapour by thousands of percent. Many people are unaware of the fact that they grind or clench their teeth during the night and this too enhances the release of mercury vapour. Put simply, if you chew gum – stop – and if you grind your teeth get a night guard (bite splint) from your dentist which may help to reduce vapour release until such time as you may be able to systematically replace your amalgam fillings.

Forms of Mercury

Part of the reason that mercury is so damaging to biological systems can be attributed to the fact that it can exist in many different forms – all of which are toxic and all of which have different properties. Many processes within the body can convert one form to another and this enables the mercury to slip through the various 'barriers' of the body and then convert within these compartments, preventing removal. The mercury is stored according to genetic predisposition, any powerful emotions being experienced and the nutrients available. All the different types of mercury exhibit different toxic effects within the various compartments of the body and this process accounts for the myriad different symptoms of toxicity.

Mercury is unique amongst metals in being a liquid at room temperature and has been given the symbol Hg which is derived from the Greek word hydragyros, meaning silver water. In its pure elemental form, the mercury atom has a full complement of electrons, including two in its outer shell, and this is expressed as Hg^0 or Hg(0). This form is a bit unstable which means that the atom readily donates one electron to form *monovalent* mercury (Hg^+ or Hg(I)), or two electrons to form *divalent* mercury (Hg^{2+} or Hg(II)), and this process is known as oxidation. In both its monovalent and divalent forms it can combine with inorganic elements such as sulphur or chlorine to form *mercurous* salts and in its divalent form it can combine with organic (carbon-containing) substances to form *mercuric* compounds.

Metallic or Elemental Mercury

Liquid mercury readily vaporizes at room or body temperature and both the tiny droplets of mercury that form on high-copper amalgams and the vapour given off amalgam fillings are examples of mercury in its pure elemental form. It is not thought to be well absorbed if swallowed, but is highly irritant and damaging to the gastrointestinal tract. It also has a very short half-life, believed to be about 10 seconds in circulation. However, the mercury vapour off-gassed from amalgam fillings has direct access to the brain through the perforated cribriform plate in the roof of the nose which permits the sense of smell. Elemental mercury is fat soluble and so mercury vapour that has penetrated the skull in this way can readily breach the blood–brain barrier and adversely affect the adjacent cluster of nerve endings that is the hypothalamus. In this form mercury can also cross the placental barrier to profoundly affect the growth and development of the foetus. The vast majority of exposure for most, however, is believed to be absorbed as vapour in the lungs from where it can pass into the red blood cells of the circulation and be converted into mercurous forms which may prove resistant to removal. The fat-soluble swallowed vapour and droplets are also absorbed into the extensive network of lymphatic vessels intended for the absorption of dietary fats and ultimately join the circulation. Mercury vapour is also driven into the tissues of the mouth as a result of the galvanic action mentioned previously and then binds tightly to the proteins of the mucosa. Elemental mercury can also readily react with exogenous substances such as the fluorine in toothpaste or the chlorine in water and also with endogenous substances such as the hydrochloric acid of the stomach to form mercurous salts.

Inorganic Mercurous Salts

Amalgam readily forms mercurous corrosion products which are abraded, swallowed and absorbed into the circulation in the intestine, from where they are routed to the liver in the portal vein to join the general circulation. These salts are toxic and corrosive and, because they are water soluble, exist mostly within the water compartments of the body such as the extracellular fluid. The body attempts to excrete these salts in the urine, leading to rapid and significant kidney damage. This form has poor fat solubility which means that it cannot cross cell membranes or the blood–brain barrier but can disrupt the structure and metabolic pathways of the cell and cause gastrointestinal damage. Various intracellular enzyme systems can also convert elemental mercury into persistent inorganic forms within tissues such as the brain and red blood cells. In the same way as the bacteria in contaminated waters can convert elemental mercury into inorganic mercury and also convert this form into the most toxic and persistent organic mercury, so can the mass of friendly bacteria in our bowels. These forms are then absorbed into both the circulation and the massive nerve plexus of the intestines, causing the digestive problems that are so familiar to FRS sufferers. In its ionic form, mercury (Hg^+ and Hg^{2+}) can be 'mistaken' by the body for other mineral ions such as sodium (Na^+) and incorporated into the active site of enzymes, thus inactivating enzyme pathways in the liver. Alternatively it may be 'mistaken' for zinc (Zn^{2+}) and incorporated into the prostate gland, for instance, causing prostate enlargement.

Organic Mercuric Compounds

There are a large number of these organomercurial compounds, however, methyl mercury (CH_3Hg^+) is the most significant mercury compound in terms of health and the environment and exists as a salt such as methyl mercuric chloride (CH_3HgCl). Mercury in this form is unfortunately extremely stable (it has a half-life of 27 years in the central nervous system), binds very firmly to sulphhydryl groups in proteins and is between *50 and 100 times more toxic* than in its elemental form. The mercuric form is less water soluble than the mercurous form but can enter all cells by dissolving in the fats that comprise the majority of the cell membrane. Once within the cell, it can be converted by enzyme systems to its mercurous form which can then not pass back through the membrane and so mercury collects within the tissues. The mercuric form is known to particularly accumulate in organelle membranes, especially those of the lysosomes (the 'suicide bags') which rupture, releasing their hydrolytic enzymes into the cell causing cell damage and possibly cell death. It also preferentially attaches to the membranes of the mitochondria, inhibiting the vital energy-producing enzyme systems of the body – with devastating results. Before organic mercury can be dislodged and transported from these binding sites, it has first to be converted into its mercurous, water-soluble form using an antioxidant such as vitamin C.

Another form of organic mercury is ethyl mercury and the body metabolizes the thimerosal used as a vaccine preservative into this form. In this way, the average child in the USA will have been exposed to an estimated 185mcg of mercury in the vaccination programme alone in recent decades. These organic mercuric forms are readily absorbed by the gastrointestinal tract and being highly fat soluble they accumulate in the brain, kidney, liver, skin and endocrine organs and can cross both the blood–brain and placental barriers. The liver also attempts to detoxify some forms of mercury via the methylation pathway in the liver and this inadvertently results in conversion of less toxic forms of mercury into the *most toxic methyl mercury* form. Anyone with mercury toxicity will have exhausted supplies of the nutrients required by this pathway and symptoms include stagnation of bile and/or the formation of gallstones and possibly cancer. In women, depletion of this pathway will also cause excess oestrogen build-up which may manifest as PMS, breast lumps and/or continued breast growth. The vast majority of methyl mercury is excreted with fats in the bile and if the processes of digestion are compromised this may lead to *significant reabsorption* in the enterohepatic circulation (the bile loop). Finally and significantly, methyl mercury is known to bind to the oestrogen receptors in females, resulting in women accumulating *twice* as much body burden of mercury as males.

The Effects of Mercury Toxicity

The first system affected by mercury toxicity is the immune system where the number of natural killer cells are reduced and thus become unable to police tumours and virus-infected cells. Various yeasts and bacteria such as Candida albicans and Escherichia coli are known to have the protective capacity to convert inorganic mercury into methyl mercury. When the immune neutrophils engulf these mercury-laden organisms they are disabled, losing both their motility and effectiveness. In this manner mercury toxicity can promote the overgrowth of yeasts which can ultimately become systemic, invading every organ and system. Intervention using antibiotics may unwittingly inflame this scenario as they obliterate the friendly bacteria controlling yeast growth – although this may not be apparent until months or years later. The affected neutrophils inevitably die as a result of consuming the mercury toxic yeasts and are dismantled in the liver where the mercury may effectively concentrate. Mercury toxicity also increases the ratios of T helper cells (which initiate an immune response) to T suppressor cells (which terminate an immune response) and this may lead to the development of allergies.

Significantly, mercury combines with the 'bar code' (the major histocompatibility complex) on the cell membrane that identifies cells as being 'self' and in so doing changes the bar code to 'non-self'. This results in the immune system attacking body cells as in the autoimmune diseases such as multiple sclerosis, Parkinson's disease, diabetes and Hashimoto's thyroiditis.

Methyl mercury also prevents cell division and generation and interferes with the formation of the structural tubulin in the microtubules of the cell and neurones and the formation of the insulating myelin sheaths around nerves. These factors, when combined with the lipophilic (fat-loving) and neurophilic (nerve-loving) nature of methyl mercury, explain the devastating and long-lasting effects both in the developing foetus and child (where tissues are growing rapidly) and in the tremors and psychological and behavioural effects in the adult. Mercury profoundly impacts the management of fats in the body too, altering steroid and cholesterol regulation and destroying and oxidizing both essential fatty acids and the phospholipids of the cell membrane. Mercury toxicity may promote elevated blood cholesterol levels (which may be protective) and ultimately cardiovascular problems. Therefore, seeking to lower cholesterol levels is treating a symptom rather than the silent and unseen cause.

Mercury also affects the mitochondria which, if deprived of adequate oxygen, switch to anaerobic energy production with the associated build-up of lactic acid which causes the muscle stiffness and aching that are familiar to most FRS sufferers. The mitochondria become unable to recycle the spent ADP back to ATP efficiently as mercury disables a key enzyme and this results in further breakdown within the cytosol into adenosine mono-phosphate (AMP) which is then excreted in the urine. It then takes up to four days to synthesize 'new' ATP from glucose and this may account for the post-exertional malaise.

Even the proponents of the use of mercury in dentistry admit that elevated amounts remain detectable in the blood for *up to three months* after an amalgam filling is either removed or placed. This is because organic mercury has a half-life in circulation of approximately 72 days and inorganic mercury a half-life of approximately 40 days. What this means is that half the original amount of organic mercury is found in circulation after 72 days and a quarter at 144 days and so on. The presumption has always been that it took this long to excrete, but we now know that possibly relatively little of the mercury is eliminated and that most of it is stored deep within body compartments like nervous tissue, body fat and cellulite, joints, the uterus in women and the sinuses in men. Dr Murray Vimy and his researchers at the University of Calgary demonstrated the rapid spread of radioactive mercury from newly placed amalgam fillings to many different organs and tissues in both sheep and monkeys. They also demonstrated a *50 per cent reduction in kidney function within a month* of amalgam placement. This means, as they stated, that you are effectively functioning with one kidney after your first amalgam filling is placed! This may indicate that the primary method of excretion in the urine becomes overwhelmed, damaging the delicate mechanisms concerned and compromising further detoxification. In 2001, researchers at the Catholic University of Rome found that patients with congestive heart failure had hugely elevated mercury levels in their hearts and Soviet experiments carried out in the 1970s also confirmed high levels of mercury in the heart and its valves. Mercury also binds to the iron-binding sites of haemoglobin, thus reducing the oxygen-carrying capacity of the blood by half, causes rupture of red blood cells and damages blood vessels, and these factors mean that the organs and tissues of the body are then not adequately oxygenated. Alzheimer's patients at autopsy also showed high levels of both mercury and lead in their brains and the expressionless face of the Alzheimer's victim may relate to mercury toxicity of the nervous supply to the facial muscles effectively causing paralysis. So it appears that mercury can be stored in almost any tissue or organ and can affect all body systems in addition to causing massive free radical damage and promoting inflammation through the release of signalling molecules known as cytokines. Figure 7 shows some of the recognized effects of mercury toxicity on the various organ systems. Intriguingly, there appears to be an inverse relationship between neurological conditions and cancer which troubles researchers but may be dependent upon the inherited predisposition of the individual to store toxins. To establish the likely extent of mercury toxicity as a causative factor in your FRS, please complete the questionnaire in figure 8.

Figure 7: The symptoms of mercury toxicity

Central nervous system
Anxiety; apathy; brain fog; depression; poor memory; poor concentration; inability to make decisions; loss of intelligence; mood swings and dark moods; outbursts of anger or rage; inappropriate emotional responses; obsessions; frequent infatuations; headaches – especially after eating; insomnia; timidness; withdrawal; passivity; clumsiness; messiness and cluttering; addictions; obsessive/compulsive behaviour; bipolar disorder; psychotic behaviour; schizophrenia; deviant behaviour; constant death wish or suicidal intent; dementia; multiple sclerosis; amyotrophic lateral sclerosis and Alzheimer's disease.

Peripheral nervous system
Numbness, tingling, tremors or pain in the head, hands and feet; twitching of the face or other muscles; loss of pain sensation and ultimately multiple sclerosis.

Gastrointestinal system
Affects the mouth causing bleeding gums; excess salivation; oral inflammation; burning mouth; lichen planus and/or leukoplakia (white patches in the mouth and cheeks); geographical tongue (continent-like 'bald' patches on the tongue); a blue gum line; amalgam 'tattoos'; a metallic taste; trigeminal neuralgia and loss of teeth. Also affects the entire digestive system causing: heartburn; bloating; poor digestion; ulcers; constipation; diarrhoea; weight gain/loss; poor appetite and excessive thirst.

Endocrine system
Typically decreases function, especially of the pituitary and hypothalamus glands, which between them regulate all the other endocrine glands. Also particularly affects the thyroid (poor metabolism and repair), adrenal glands (poor stress response), pancreas (poor blood sugar control) and the gonads.

Immune system
Alters ratio of helper to suppressor T lymphocytes causing both a suppressed and overactive immune response. Suppression leads to chronic, recurrent or frequent viral, bacterial or fungal infections, especially Candida and, ultimately, cancer. An overactive or 'confused' immune system leads to hypersensitivity and allergies. Changes coding on cells inducing autoimmune diseases.

Lymphatic system
Causes stagnation of the lymphatic circulation and creates toxic lymph leading to swelling of extremities such as the ankles, hands and face; swollen tonsils and sore throat.

A Generational Issue

Fertility

Amalgam has been used for several generations now and the problems that occult mercury toxicity is creating are becoming more serious with each generation. First, many women carrying a large body burden of toxic metals are either unable to get pregnant or take a pregnancy to term, or produce babies with birth defects and metal toxicity. Men, too, are affected as sperm become unable to swim effectively, are reduced in number and contain DNA damage that can give rise to birth defects. Male fertility has dropped suddenly and precipitously in recent years. Sperm counts are now *half* of those in 1940 and have dropped by a *third* in a decade, and increased alcohol consumption, xeno-oestrogens (including toxic metals) and pesticides are the main suspects.

Figure 7: cont.

Cardiovascular system
Chest pains, irregular heartbeat and palpitations; high blood pressure; raised cholesterol and 'Syndrome X'.

Respiratory system
Asthma and breathlessness.

Skin
Rashes; excessive itching; excessive sweating; eczema; alopecia; cold hands and feet even in moderate or warm weather; the face, palms of the hands and soles of the feet frequently are red, have a rash or shed skin; acrodynia (pink disease) causes redness of the skin; grey hair; loss of hair and/or nails.

Ear, nose and throat
Various problems including recurrent infections; deafness; poor balance; tinnitus; dizziness and sinusitis.

Eyes
Causes macular degeneration; dim vision; difficulty focusing and deteriorating eyesight.

Reproductive system
In women: uterine fibroids; menstrual cycle disturbances; infertility; miscarriage; difficulties of pregnancy; birth defects. Mercury passes to the developing foetus in the umbilicus and to the nursing baby in the breast milk. In men: premature ejaculation; enlarged prostate gland; impotence; sperm are abnormal, reduced in number and non-motile causing infertility.

Musculoskeletal system
Constant or frequent muscle and joint pains; back pain; frequent leg cramps; arthritis and temperomandibular joint (TMJ) dysfunction; difficulty standing up; atrophy of muscles; leg tremors and muscle weakness (especially in women).

Urinary system
Incontinence (especially in women); bedwetting in children and difficulty with urination in men; frequent urination; burning sensation upon urination/cystitis; kidney damage.

General
Low body temperature; fatigue; premature ageing and unexplained fluid retention; fainting or feeling faint.

Pregnancy

As a rule, the later in life the first pregnancy, the more opportunity the mother will have had to accumulate a significant toxic burden. A woman is thought to pass up to two-thirds of this load to her unborn child. Part of the mechanism is that methyl mercury is able to cross the placental barrier and binds to the developing foetus's blood more tightly than to the mother's blood. The foetus has no independent means of excretion until it is born and so typically the baby has two to three times the mercury levels of the mother. To appreciate the significance of this process, consider that these toxins are being incorporated into the deepest and most sensitive tissues of the developing foetus and being concentrated twenty-fold as they are passed from a 65kg (140lb) woman to a 3kg (7lb) baby. As a consequence, the level of mercury in the brain of her baby is *directly proportional to the number of amalgam fillings in the mother's mouth.*

Figure 8: Mercury toxicity questionnaire

Instructions: Tick every question to which the answer is yes and total.

1.   Do you have CFS, ME, fibromyalgia or an autoimmune disease? ☐
2.   Do you suffer with a profound fatigue that is not relieved by rest? ☐
3.   Do you constantly or frequently feel cold? ☐
4.   Do you frequently feel hot or cold when others are comfortable? ☐
5.   Do you have unexplained and markedly different 'good' and 'bad' days? ☐
6.   Do you get frequent headaches and/or migranes? ☐
7.   Do you suffer from persistent or chronic insomnia? ☐
8.   Are you frequently drowsy and/or feel the need to sleep during the day? ☐
9.   Have you gained or lost weight without significant changes in your diet? ☐
10. Do you frequently feel tired, weak or shaky just a few hours after eating? ☐
11. Do you struggle to focus or does your ability to focus change during the day? ☐
12. Has your colour vision deteriorated? ☐
13. Do you have poor night vision? ☐
14. Do you sometimes have difficulty moving your eyes? ☐
15. Is your balance poor and/or do you frequently feel dizzy? ☐
16. Is your hearing poor? ☐
17. Is it difficult to distinguish conversation over background noise? ☐
18. Do you have difficulty making sense of what you hear? ☐
19. Do you have tinnitus (ringing in the ears)? ☐
20. Do you have a poor sense of smell? ☐
21. Was your puberty unusually early or late? ☐
22. Do you have a history of infertility? ☐
23. Is your libido poor or non-existent? ☐
24. Do you need to urinate frequently or urgently? ☐
25. Do you get up in the night to urinate more than once? ☐
26. Do you persistently or frequently have a sore throat? ☐
27. Do you have multiple chemical sensitivities? ☐
28. Do you suffer with allergies? ☐
29. Do you suffer with chronic, recurrent or frequent infections? ☐
30. Do you have frequent or recurrent athlete's foot, 'jock itch', thrush or cystitis? ☐
31. Do you have difficulty making decisions? ☐
32. Do you have trouble concentrating? ☐
33. Has your intelligence diminished? ☐
34. Do you have a poor memory? ☐
35. Do you experience difficulty finding the right words? ☐
36. Does it require a great effort to think clearly? ☐
37. Do you have trouble multitasking? ☐
38. Do you have difficulty articulating words? ☐
39. Do you have difficulty writing or doing tasks which require fine motor skills? ☐
40. Are you clumsy and/or accident prone? ☐
41. Do you have asthma or bronchitis? ☐
42. Are you sensitive to tobacco smoke, petrol (gasoline) or paint fumes? ☐
43. Do you get breathless easily? ☐
44. Have you been told that you have particularly bad breath on occasions? ☐
45. Does your heart occasionally race or hammer for no reason? ☐
46. Do you have chest pains and/or angina? ☐
47. Do you have either a slow/rapid heart rate or high/low blood pressure? ☐
48. Do you have raised blood cholesterol levels? ☐
49. Do you frequently feel faint? ☐
50. Do you suffer with water retention (often affecting the legs)? ☐
51. Do you have bleeding gums and/or tender or mobile teeth? ☐
52. Do you occasionally get a metallic taste in your mouth? ☐
53. Do you get mouth ulcers? ☐
54. Do you have an inflamed or burning mouth? ☐
55. Do you have any bald or white patches on your cheeks or tongue? ☐
56. Do you suffer with diarrhoea and/or constipation? ☐

Figure 8: cont.

57. Do you frequently have abdominal discomfort and pain? ❏
58. Have you lost your appetite? ❏
59. Do you tend to be very thirsty? ❏
60. Do you have food intolerances (especially dairy and gluten)? ❏
61. Do you have extremely dry, itchy skin, eczema or psoriasis? ❏
62. Do you either sweat profusely/get night sweats or are you unable to sweat at all? ❏
63. Does your sweat have an unusual cloying smell sometimes? ❏
64. Do you bruise easily? ❏
65. Do you frequently have cold hands and feet? ❏
66. Do you have peeling skin on your hands, feet or ankles? ❏
67. Do you have a puffy face or inflamed or flaky skin around your eyes? ❏
68. Do you have a build-up of dry skin on your hands and/or feet? ❏
69. Do you occasionally get a pricking, fizzing or stabbing sensation in your skin? ❏
70. Do you have any red colouration of your skin which may worsen when wet? ❏
71. Do you have weak nails that tear or flake easily? ❏
72. Have you currently or historically lost any underarm, pubic, leg or head hair? ❏
73. Is the quality of your hair poor and/or has the quality of your hair deteriorated? ❏
74. Would you describe yourself as anxious or depressed? ❏
75. Would you describe yourself as shy or withdrawn and easily embarrassed? ❏
76. Are you easily angered, irritated or upset? ❏
77. Are you inclined to indulge in obsessive or compulsive thoughts or behaviours? ❏
78. Does life seem an endless, joyless struggle? ❏
79. Do you lack motivation and feel apathetic? ❏
80. Are you easily overwhelmed or discouraged? ❏
81. Do you seem to have upset others without understanding why? ❏
82. Do you handle stress poorly? ❏
83. Do you experience unexplained mood swings or have dark or suicidal moods? ❏
84. Do you suffer with TMJ (jaw joint) dysfunction? ❏
85. Do you have constant or frequent joint pain(s) and/or arthritis? ❏
86. Do you have constant or frequent muscle pains? ❏
87. Do you have any muscle tremors? ❏
88. Do you have poor exercise tolerance? ❏
89. Do you frequently get cramps in your legs? ❏
90. Do your muscles tire easily? ❏
91. Do you suffer with any tics or twitches – especially of facial muscles? ❏
92. Do you have restless legs at night? ❏
93. Is it particularly difficult to stand up? ❏

Women Only:
94. Do you have a history of heavy, missed or irregular periods? ❏
95. Do you have a history of miscarriages and/or still births? ❏
96. Do you have severe period pains and/or PMT? ❏
97. Does your vagina and/or vulva occasionally or persistently feel raw or sore? ❏
98. Does your menstrual bleed have a brown colouration? ❏
99. Do you have uterine fibroids? ❏
100. Do you occasionally or persistently suffer with urinary (stress) incontinence? ❏

Men Only:
94. Do you occasionally or persistently suffer with impotence? ❏
95. Do you occasionally or persistently suffer with premature ejaculation? ❏
96. Do you occasionally or persistently experience difficulty urinating? ❏

Interpreting the results:

Likely Degree of Mercury Toxicity	Women	Men
Some mercury toxicity	1–19	1–15
Mild mercury toxicity	20–39	16–35
Moderate mercury toxicity	40–59	36–55
Severe mercury toxicity	60–79	56–75
Mercury poisoning	80–100	76–96

These babies are often born with mercury incorporated into their brain stems, which may manifest as ADHD, ADD, autism, hyperactivity, dyslexia or dyspraxia. Alarmingly, but perhaps not surprisingly, newborn babies test to an *average* of 287 circulating toxins at birth and one study found that an analysis of the levels of just *5 toxic metals* predicted learning disabilities with almost total accuracy.

However, mercury may affect other organ systems and the phenomenal rise in the incidence of asthma in the young may be another consequence possibly of the adrenal glands being adversely affected *in utero*. The male sex hormone, testosterone, is thought to compound mercury toxicity in the developing child and the female sex hormone, oestrogen, is thought to provide some protection. It is these two factors combined that account for the fact that boys are four times more likely than girls to be autistic. Boys are also more likely to be affected if they are the first born, which lends further support to the toxic load theory. The symptoms of autism may manifest in the toddler rather than the newborn because the in-born toxic load slowly allows the overgrowth of microbes and the toxins they produce. Alternatively or additionally, the increased toxic load of the vaccination programme may tip some vulnerable babies and children past the point of no return. The full scale of the problem may not yet be apparent, however one-quarter of American children are now classed as behaviourally or developmentally abnormal. The potentially lifelong plight of those damaged both in terms of compromised IQ and their ability to function and earn combined with the loss and costs to both their families and society is almost unthinkable.

Second and subsequent children may get off more lightly depending upon how long a gap there was between pregnancies, whether toxin stores were replenished generally and whether any amalgam fillings were removed or replaced. The University of Calgary team found that radioactive mercury from amalgams inserted into the teeth of pregnant sheep was found to accumulate particularly in the liver and pituitary gland of the young at a higher level than that of the mother. This transmission is now recognized and the placing of dental amalgam fillings during pregnancy has been discouraged. For this reason, if you are either already pregnant or likely to become pregnant during treatment, *you should not undertake the metal detoxification outlined in this book or indeed any detoxification programme.* Remember also the extended half-life of mercury and ensure that you allow several months to elapse between the end of any detoxification regime and becoming pregnant. However, the more toxic metals and toxins generally that both you and your partner can remove before you attempt to become pregnant, the greater the chances of conception and a healthy baby. For women this issue is more significant than for men because whilst the father contributes one (admittedly very important) cell to the process, the mother contributes all the raw materials to make a little human being.

Breastfeeding

Breastfeeding should be sacrosanct and essential for priming the baby's immune system. However, because both breast tissue and the breast milk it produces are high in fats, mercury and other toxins such as phthalates and flame retardants (PBDEs) preferentially accumulate in the milk. One study showed that concentrations of mercury in breast milk were eight times higher than in the mother's blood and in another study one in ten of the mothers had breast milk so toxic that it should have been treated as toxic waste! *For this reason, you should also not undertake any detoxification whilst breastfeeding.*

The Future

Given the absolutely monumental scale of the problem facing us, is it any wonder that the authorities seem keen to hold the official line on mercury toxicity? Others, such as the toxicologist Alan Stern, who contributed to the Unites States National Research Council report on mercury toxicity, seem less sure. He was quoted as saying, 'It's really unclear what's going on with dental amalgams. It's a snake pit and the issue is complicated by the potential for panic and lawsuits.' Both Canada and the USA have ongoing class action lawsuits relating to mercury toxicity, reminiscent of the huge previous tobacco and asbestosis suits. Any admission or settlement could possibly bankrupt a country and certainly an organization such as the National Health Service in the United Kingdom. Some countries such as Japan, Russia, Sweden, Denmark, Austria, Norway and Germany have partial or total bans on the use of dental amalgam and some US states now require warnings to be posted and/or that the patient makes an informed decision about the risks. Dental amalgam almost certainly would not pass any safety tests were it to be introduced today. Degussa, the German dental materials manufacturer, has ceased production of dental amalgam in spite of the fact that it was responsible for 50 per cent of their annual turnover (citing other reasons). Given the mounting crippling personal and societal costs of degenerative and serious illness, ought we not adopt the precautionary principle and – in the words of the Hippocratic Oath – 'Do no harm'?

Don't hold your breath though. Where big money and vested interests are concerned, one only needs look at the tobacco industry to see how long it took for the 'experts' to decide that smoking was undeniably a cause of cancer and lung disease. Tens of thousands of young British servicemen exposed to huge amounts of radiation in atomic bomb trials in the Pacific fifty years ago are currently still fighting for compensation as the damage to both them and their offspring has become apparent as the years unfold. The UK Ministry of Defence disputes the claim and probably intends to do so until most of the affected personnel are dead. At the time of writing, the US Food and Drug Administration and the American Dental Association have both recently taken down reassuring statements from their websites about the use of mercury in dental amalgam and the Center for Disease Control has recently deleted an entire webpage refuting amalgam as a cause of serious illness. They know that they are staring down the barrel of the biggest legal action in history – they are just hoping they will be retired by the time the smelly stuff hits the fan. The moral of this story is: Think for yourself. There are huge vested interests at work and not one of them is ultimately interested in you or your health. As a parent, too, you have a sacred duty to protect your children – irrespective of what some official (who may or may not be worthy of the trust invested in them) may determine is in their best interests. However, please read on before rushing to the phone to make your dental appointment!

Chapter 10
Endocrine Disorders

One or more elements of the endocrine system are invariably affected in fatigue-related syndromes and are an integral part of the disorder. This chapter examines the most common endocrine disorders.

The Endocrine System Uncovered

In the mid-20th century, a young medical researcher called Dr Hans Selye categorized the stages of response to chronic stress in what he called the General Adaptation Syndrome. He identified this as largely involving the endocrine glands and forming the common pathway to sickness after which one or more organs or systems would fail resulting in a diagnosable illness (according to the dictates of allopathic medicine). When first placed under stress he found that the body responded with a heightened 'fight or flight' reaction which he called an *alarm* state. If the organism survives this acute state, then it will adapt to chronic stress by up-regulating the endocrine system in what Dr Selye called the *resistance* stage. This stage is intended to be a temporary survival mechanism and cannot be sustained indefinitely, and if the stressor is removed during this stage the organism can still spontaneously recover. Eventually, however, all adaptive mechanisms fail and this leads to the rapid onset of an *exhaustion* state. At this point the organism cannot recover without sustained and purposeful intervention.

Endocrine Dysfunction and FRS

> What we feel and think and are is to a great extent determined by the state of our ductless glands and viscera.
>
> **Aldous Huxley**

You will not be surprised to learn that all FRS sufferers have reached this exhaustion state and as a result may have a wide range of distressing and perplexing symptoms relating to endocrine dysfunction. It can be very difficult at this stage to tease out the various elements and these disorders often go undiagnosed by allopathic medical methods for a wide variety of reasons (see also chapter 5). In this chapter, we will examine the most commonly found endocrine issues which relate to the thyroid and adrenal glands, pancreas, gonads and master glands in the brain. There is often a family history of endocrine disorders, which may have gone undiagnosed or been wrongly diagnosed. So as you refer to the signs and symptoms of these disorders, consider whether other family members – alive or deceased – have manifested any of these symptoms.

The Causes of Endocrine Dysfunction

There are several possible causes of endocrine problems generally including:

- Food intolerances – most commonly to gluten (in most grains) and/or dairy products
- Consuming foods known as goitrogens which can damage the thyroid gland
- Exposure to environmental and occupational toxins
- Mineral deficiencies
- The use of synthetic hormones (the contraceptive pill, HRT) or steroids
- Exposure to ionizing radiation, electromagnetic radiation or 'dirty' electricity
- Toxic metals which bind to the hormone receptors in the tissues preventing docking and also replace the essential mineral in the hormone, altering its 3D shape and rendering it ineffective. Toxic metals also block mineral receptors and promote the overgrowth of Candida within the endocrine glands.

Thyroid Gland Disorders

The thyroid gland is extremely sensitive and is often the first target of 'autoimmunity' (mercury toxicity) and may also be the last to recover. The thyroid gland can become overactive (hyperthyroidism) and signs of this include an increased metabolic rate, anxiety, restlessness, hair loss, heart palpitations and weight loss in spite of a good appetite. However, by far the most common problem found in FRS is that of an underactive thyroid gland which is also known as hypothyroidism (where 'hypo-' means low) or myxoedema ('myx-' refers to mucous and '-oedema' to swelling). Sometimes a mixed picture can present with a struggling gland alternating between these two extremes before finally failing. Occasionally, because the thyroid gland has two lobes, one can be underactive and the other lobe can be endeavouring to compensate, leading to a mixed picture until failure finally becomes inevitable. For the signs and symptoms associated with hypothyroidism please refer to figure 9. Please

Figure 9: The signs and symptoms of hypothyroidism

Skin, hair and nails

Pale, dry, itchy skin; cracked skin on heels and hands; psoriasis; eczema; red/orange skin (especially the soles of the feet and the palms of the hands); decreased sweating. Dry, coarse, brittle hair; loss of hair including underarm or pubic hair; loss of the outer third of the eyebrow (Hertog's sign); flaky nails that split easily and that often lack half-moons.

Musculosketal system

More frequent and severe muscle cramps; muscle stiffness; rheumatoid-type joint pain; joint stiffness; large calf muscles; carpal tunnel syndrome; feet may continue to grow in size.

Nervous system

Pins and needles and/or numbness.

Immune system

Poor immune response; frequent and/or chronic infections; prolonged healing.

Genitourinary system

In females: cessation of periods; sparse periods; profuse, heavy and/or irregular periods; miscarriages, stillbirth or infertility; worsening PMT. In both sexes: non-existent libido and loss of sexual responsiveness; nocturnal incontinence in children.

Cardiovascular system

Slow heart rate; slightly elevated blood pressure; elevated cholesterol level; elevated homocysteine level; palpitations.

Respiratory system

Breathlessness; feeling that there is a lump in the throat (swollen thyroid gland); a hoarse voice; excessive production of mucous; snoring.

Special senses

Hearing and/or balance problems; tinnitus; reduced night vision.

Digestive system

Constipation and/or diarrhoea; IBS; loss of appetite; alcohol intolerance; dairy intolerance often found.

Mental/psychological symptoms

Slow thinking and comprehending; forgetfulness; worsening problems with memory; difficulty stringing words together. Depression; sadness; melancholy; pessimism; lack of confidence; anger; irritability; not caring about anything; crying easily; mood swings; anxiety; panic attacks; hallucinations; paranoid, suicidal and morbid thoughts.

Miscellaneous

An overtly swollen thyroid 'goitre' (a fat neck that often forms defined creases); feeling cold and also not handling heat well; shaking; headaches or migraines; insomnia, or sleeping heavily and waking exhausted; tendency to fall asleep during the day; exhaustion, lethargy and weariness; everything is an effort – 'like walking through treacle'; clumsiness and lack of coordination. Weight gain; difficulty losing weight; puffiness especially of the ankles, hands and face; puffy eyelids possibly with prominent bags below the eyes. Suspected link to breast cancer.

consider whether you have experienced any of these signs either in the present or historically. There appears to be a particular propensity for thyroid problems in people with Celtic ancestry for reasons that are not fully understood.

It is worth noting here that for some reason, whilst doctors in mainland Europe apparently check for low blood pressure as much as they check for high blood pressure, in the UK and USA this appears to be a bit of a blind spot. I had a pulse rate of approximately 40 beats per minute for as long as I can remember and this always met with approval from the dozens of doctors and nurses who measured it over the decades rather than being seen as an overt sign of hypothyroidism. It might have been regarded as an indication of a fantastically efficient cardiovascular system in a top-flight athlete, but as should have been evident, this was not the case with me. This meant that my heart was beating *43,000 times less per day* than it should have been and this obviously has huge implications for perfusion and oxygenation of the entire body – and especially the brain. Hypothyroidism also causes stagnation of bile in the liver and constipation, and these factors too have profound knock-on effects upon all organs and systems.

DIY Tests for Hypothyroidism

If you identify with several of the symptoms listed in figure 9, then it is worth doing a few simple tests yourself that might help to indicate whether an underactive thyroid gland is an issue for you before going to see the doctor.

The Barnes Temperature Test

Most people with hypothyroidism have a low metabolic rate and a correspondingly low body temperature. This technique involves taking a reading of the lowest temperature first thing in the morning and was originally developed by Dr Broda Barnes, for which reason this test is sometimes named after her. Use an electric thermometer under your tongue and have it ready next to the bed, do not move about at all before taking the reading and do not use an electric blanket. If you are a menstruating woman, then this should be done on days two to four of your period. You may also wish to take your temperature later in the day for comparison. Take a few readings and average them out and check others to make sure the thermometer is working accurately also. A normal average basal temperature is 36.6–36.8°C (97.8–98.2°F) and a normal daytime temperature is 37–37.2°C (98.6–99.0°F) and the lower the reading the greater the hypothyroidism. Be aware that any infection or even candidal overgrowth in the intestines may elevate a normally low body temperature. Conversely, this is a good way to monitor your improvement. You may feel you do not need to use a thermometer. You already know that you feel cold all the time and may have cold extremities much of the time too.

Heart Rate/Blood Pressure

You can buy a blood pressure/heart rate monitor cheaply these days and use it to check your blood pressure and heart rate. An average blood pressure reading should be about 120/80mmHg. The higher of these two readings tells you what the peak pressure is in your arteries when your heart is contracting and the lower reading shows what the blood pressure falls to between heart contractions. With hypothyroidism blood pressures can be raised or normal, but are often lowered and there is reduced pulse pressure – i.e. the difference between the two readings will be reduced – for example to 110/85mmHg. Normal values for blood pressure rise with age and the average value for older people is 140/90mmHg. Take several readings at rest, whilst sitting upright, and keep your wrist at heart level and then average them. Do not take readings immediately after a meal, unless you wish to establish food intolerances (see chapter 14). A normal pulse is 72 beats per minute. Any significant deviation from this indicates possible thyroid dysfunction with the pulse being slowed in hypothyroidism and more rapid in hyperthyroidism. My observation is that blood pressure tends to rise as the heart rate falls in order to maintain perfusion of the organs and that the heart rate is very much a function of thyroxine levels and thyroid health.

Use Your Eyes

Hypothyroidism has a very characteristic look with heaviness of the face – especially the eyes – and possibly a fat neck that forms folds. Look back on old photographs and compare them. Those with hypothyroidism also tend to have an enlarged tongue with impressions of the teeth in the sides and this is something you can check in the mirror. The soles of the feet and palms of the hands often have an orange/red colouration due to betacarotene build-up; the outer third of the eyebrow thins or is lost and the fingernails are weak and may lack half-moons.

The Problems with Blood Tests Assessing Thyroid Function

Health consists of having the same diseases as one's neighbours.

Quentin Crisp

If you think that you may be hypothyroid and you have either never been tested, or have not been tested recently, then it is worthwhile approaching your doctor and asking for a blood test. However, be warned that blood tests often come back as 'within normal limits' in spite of the individual quite obviously having an underactive thyroid and the reasons for this are detailed below.

- The normal ranges are determined by testing people presumed to be healthy and then regarding the middle 90 per cent of test values as representing the 'normal' range. The problem with this approach is that up to one in three adults are estimated to have an underactive thyroid gland, with the general population being affected to a lesser extent. This is probably because of the universal nature of toxicity in general and mercury toxicity in particular, and skews the reference ranges which, possibly as a result, have been revised downwards in recent years.

- There is a huge amount of individual variation between people, so what you need to know is what *your* optimal thyroxine levels are, not what a population average is.

- For economic reasons, many doctors only test for thyroid stimulating hormone (TSH) which is the pituitary hormone that stimulates the thyroid to function. The assumption is that if circulating thyroxine levels are low then TSH levels will be elevated. If you do ask for a thyroid function test, then request a 'full panel' test which measures the output of the thyroid gland and whether the precursor hormones it produces are being converted into their active forms in the tissues. Specifically request that the active *free* forms of thyroxine and tri-iodothyronine (T4 and T3) be assessed in preference to total T4 and T3 levels which show hormone levels in the inactive transport form. TSH levels may also not be a good indicator of tissue levels of thyroid hormones because the pituitary gland possesses its own enzymes to convert T4 to T3, whereas elsewhere in the body this is mediated by a selenium-containing molecule which is often rendered ineffective by mercury. Even if circulating levels of hormones are determined to be 'normal', the tissue receptor sites are often blocked by toxic metals meaning that it is the *tissues that are functionally hypothyroid*, not the circulation. A thyrotropin releasing hormone (TRH) stimulation test involves assessing TSH levels before and 30 minutes after injecting the hypothalamic hormone. TRH is thought to be the most sensitive test of thyroid function. An antinuclear antibody (ANA) test may also assess the possibility of so-called 'autoimmunity'.

- The thyroid gland has a high requirement for iodine because each molecule of thyroxine (T4) contains four iodine molecules. Other similar elements such as fluorine, chlorine and toxic metals can be 'mistaken' by the body for iodine rendering the resulting T4 molecule ineffective although tests will not detect this substitution.

- A dysfunctional gland can also make so-called 'reverse T3' (rT3) or 'junk T3' which is the wrong shape to dock on the receptors, but will still show as being normal in a blood test.

- Blood samples will vary according to when they were taken because thyroxine levels fluctuate greatly over the course of the day and are also released into the circulation in a pulsatile manner, which means that levels vary over the course of an hour or so also.

- Lastly, your thyroid gland may only be minimally underfunctioning, which may be hard to detect but this effect compounds over decades.

Supplementation for Thyroid Disorders

The hormone thyroxine governs practically every activity in the body and establishing adequate circulating levels of this hormone early on in treatment is crucial to recovery. Supplementing thyroxine may be a necessary step to recovery and hopefully as you detoxify you may be able to wean yourself off this medication under supervision. Many of the symptoms of fibromyalgia in particular are relieved by thyroxine even if blood tests show circulating levels to be normal and doses required may be in excess of what most doctors would be comfortable prescribing to get relief of symptoms. Within reason, the dose that is right for you is the one that relieves your symptoms, normalizes your heart rate, blood pressure and temperature, eliminates the bright colouration of the palms of your hands and soles of your feet, stabilizes your weight and, if female and pre-menopausal, regulates your menstrual cycle to approximately every 28 days. The benefits of thyroxine may or may not be immediately obvious but compound over time and may take six months to two years to fully take effect.

If your doctor agrees that you have hypothyroidism, they will typically prescribe synthetic thyroxine. Some people, however, fail to improve because they cannot convert this into the active T3 form and for this reason some doctors are willing to supplement the thyroxine with a small amount of synthetic T3. Alternatively, Armour Thyroid is a natural combined extract of T4 and T3 from cows or pigs that, until recently, was available in the USA, and a full replacement dose is regarded as being five grains, although you should check with your doctor. However, in 2009 the FDA asked the manufacturers to make a New Drug Application and it is not known when this will be available again. As the adrenal glands fail they down-regulate the thyroid gland and supplementing thyroxine necessarily places a bigger demand upon the adrenal glands. So if you fail to feel any better, or if you actually feel worse for taking thyroxine, it is most probably because you have adrenal fatigue that also needs treating, or needs treating first. The resin of the Mukul myrrh tree, known as gum guggul, can also be supplemented to aid conversion of T4 to T3.

If the doctor's tests are 'normal' but you still think you have a problem, or if your doctor is willing to prescribe supplemental hormones but you also want to detoxify and regenerate your thyroid gland, seek the advice of a suitably trained professional with experience of these natural methods. **Note:** it is advisable to check your blood pressure and heart rate regularly throughout detoxification to dynamically monitor your thyroid function, and inform your health care practitioner of any changes.

The Emotional Meaning of Thyroid Disorders

On an emotional level, thyroid problems often have their origins around either neglectful or suffocating mothering and also in experiences of being a mother. Other issues relate to things that were not – or could not – be said, and your ability to speak your truth.

Adrenal Gland Disorders

Most people with FRS will have compromised or severely compromised adrenal function. The adrenal glands have an inner core of nervous tissue that produces adrenaline and noradrenaline (epinephrine and norephinephrine) and an outer rind that produces steroid hormones. These steroid hormones include aldosterone (which regulates electrolytes), small amounts of mostly male sex hormones (in both sexes), dehydroepiandrosterone (DHEA) and cortisol. The immediate response to stress is to produce adrenaline with cortisol providing medium-to-long-term support. A history of stress often predates or precipitates a decline into FRS and in the resistance stage of the chronic stress response the HPA axis (hypothalamus-pituitary-adrenal axis) is activated and cortisol levels may be elevated. However, in the exhaustion stage cortisol levels may be reduced and both are found in FRS sufferers. DHEA is thought to modulate the long-term cortisol response and has been referred to as the anti-ageing hormone. A frequent finding is that FRS sufferers may be able to keep going in a crisis on adrenaline (epinephrine) and then frequently collapse when the stress is over, due to lack of synthesis of cortisol. Allopathic medicine only recognizes two extreme forms of adrenal dysfunction and these are Cushing's disease (extreme excess circulating cortisol) and Addison's disease (extreme deficiency of cortisol). There is, of course, a great spectrum of shades of grey before these black and white extremes are reached. Raised levels of cortisol cause suppression of both the immune response and inflammation, and at lowered levels may fail to control an aberrant immune response and permit widespread inflammation. As a result, any condition which is improved by taking steroids in any form is probably at least partly caused by underactive adrenal glands. The HPA axis also regulates temperature, blood pressure, pulse rate, perspiration, bladder function, memory and emotion. Ultimately, the thyroid and adrenal glands tend to fail together and it can frequently be hard to determine which is the cause and which the effect.

Adrenal glands can become overactive in the resistance stage and this disorder shares many of the symptoms associated with taking steroids or Cushing's disease. Symptoms include developing a 'moonface'; thin skin with increased body hair; a 'buffalo' hump; gaining weight around the middle whilst extremities become thinner; osteoporosis and

Figure 10: The signs and symptoms of hypoadrenia

Skin, hair and nails
Pale, translucent skin; dark rings around the eyes; area(s) of excessive bronze pigmentation somewhere on the body; red fingertips; loss of either pubic or underarm hair or hair on the lower legs in men.

Musculoskeletal system
Muscle weakness leading to back or loin pain, knee or ankle problems.

Immune system
Repeated infections or poor response to infections; any inflammatory condition; allergies; being ill the first week or so of every holiday or break from work/study.

Genitourinary system
In females: menstrual disturbances; menstrual bleed stops and resumes; PMS and difficult menopause; experiencing a poor pregnancy until the third trimester (approximately 24 weeks).

Cardiovascular system
Low blood pressure (occasionally high blood pressure); haemorrhoids; varicose veins; poor exercise tolerance; fainting.

Respiratory system
Asthma; respiratory allergies; hay fever.

Digestive system
Diarrhoea; constipation or IBS.

Mental/psychological symptoms
Confusion; memory loss; depression; anxiety; irritability; feeling that something is wrong; post-natal depression; inability to concentrate. Individuals often keep going on adrenaline through stressful times (exams/house move), only to collapse afterwards due to inadequate production of cortisol.

Miscellaneous
Gaining weight around the middle without overeating; conversely being thin and weak; chronic fatigue; heat and/or cold sensitivity with cold hands and/or feet; being constantly hungry and feeling shaky 3–4 hours after eating. Input from the special senses may be intensified and pain sensitivity increased.

a tendency towards infections and high blood pressure. However, the majority of FRS sufferers have probably reached the exhaustion stage of the adaptation syndrome and have adrenal fatigue, which is also known as hypoadrenia. The signs and symptoms of adrenal fatigue are listed in figure 10 and the chances are high that if you have any of these symptoms, and especially *if they date back to a stressful event, illness or respiratory infection*, adrenal fatigue is a significant component of your FRS. Doctors tend not to look for – or recognize – adrenal fatigue until it is very severe, although veterinarians routinely test for it in ailing dogs.

Laboratory Tests for Hypoadrenia
Blood and Urine Tests

Doctors can test adrenal function with blood tests or timed collection of urine over a 24-hour period. These tests are of debatable usefulness and even if they confirm adrenal fatigue, the treatment given may be counterproductive.

Saliva Test

Samples of saliva can be collected at intervals throughout the day and tested for levels of the adrenal hormones dehydroepiandrosterone (DHEA) and cortisol. Salivary hormone levels are thought to more accurately indicate the amount of hormone *within* the cells as opposed to that in circulation and can be arranged through a naturopath or nutritionist.

DIY Tests for Hypoadrenia

Blood Pressure

The main veins in your legs have valves to prevent blood pooling there, but the large veins in the torso do not and rely upon the stress response of the adrenals to contract them in order to maintain vital blood pressure to your head. If you already have a blood pressure monitor you can try taking your blood pressure lying down and then immediately on standing up. In healthy people there will be a slight rise in systolic pressure (the higher figure) as the body overcompensates. If your blood pressure falls and takes a while to recover, this is a sign of poor adrenal function. If you routinely feel weak, shaky or faint on standing up – this is why.

Pupil Size and Response

Have someone shine a torch in your eyes in a darkened room. In a healthy person this should produce a contraction of the pupil. However, if you have adrenal fatigue, your pupils may fluctuate between contracting and dilating or may dilate because the muscles of the iris, like other muscles, rapidly fatigue. Also, because those who have reached the terminal stages of adrenal exhaustion tend to have permanently dilated pupils, ask someone to compare the size of your pupils to others.

Scratch Test

Draw a line on your belly using a blunt object. The response in someone with normal adrenal function is that the line will turn from white to red within a minute or so. In someone whose adrenal glands are fatigued the line will become whiter and spread to become diffuse white over a few minutes. If you react positively to this test it is confirmatory of adrenal fatigue, but the absence of this sign does not discount this possibility.

Supplementation for Hypoadrenia

The adrenal glands have a very high requirement for several nutrients, particularly vitamin C and the B vitamins – especially B3 and B5. The adrenal glands, too, can be nursed back to health, but this will require expert guidance. Some have found improvements by supplementing DHEA, although this appears to be of greater benefit in men than in women and is treating a symptom rather than a cause. Thyroxine increases the demands made upon the adrenal glands and so adrenal issues may need to be addressed first or contemporaneously with the thyroid.

Pancreatic Disorders

Every time we eat refined carbohydrates or sugar-containing foods or drinks, they are quickly broken down into glucose which is absorbed in the intestine and then circulates in the blood. Rises in blood sugar levels above an acceptable limit are met with a release of insulin from the pancreas. This means that new sugars are not synthesized and that circulating sugar is converted either into fat for long-term storage or glycogen (which is a more readily available form of storage) in the muscles and liver. When blood sugar levels fall below the lower acceptable limit, first glycogen and then fat are broken down under the influence of another pancreatic hormone – glucagon. Poorly controlled blood sugar levels are thought to be a common cause of depression and behavioural changes as the brain has a high requirement for, and is very sensitive to, circulating glucose.

The body was never designed for the diet that we eat today. For Stone Age man, the sweetest thing he might ever have encountered would have been a little honey or fruit and the sweetness informed him that the fruit was ripe to eat. These sugars would have been slow-releasing and have come packaged with fibre, minerals and vitamins, not the highly refined sugar products stripped of all nutrients that we know today. When our bodies detect rapidly rising blood sugar levels, they overreact in response to a source that would have been slow releasing for many millennia. This means that the body over-corrects for rises in blood sugar, leading to a corresponding low blood sugar level (hypoglycaemia) a few hours later. Poorly controlled blood sugar levels are one of the most common adrenal gland stressors. A great many people are in a vicious cycle of eating starchy, sugary foods to lift them up, only to crave more sugars and refined carbohydrates when their blood sugar levels drop precipitously a few hours later and this is the rollercoaster known as dysglycaemia. The problem is that the body develops ways of protecting the internal environment of the cell and it does this by down-regulating the number of insulin receptors on the cell membrane to prevent too much glucose entering the cell. This can lead to the paradoxical situation of having dangerously high blood glucose levels (which can cause the kind of arterial damage seen in diabetics) and yet little or no glucose *within* the cells for energy production – leading to exhaustion. This is known as insulin resistance and is a pre-diabetic state and a component of 'Syndrome X'.

Figure 11: The signs and symptoms of pancreatic dysfunction

Immune system
Overgrowth of Candida: thrush, athlete's foot, 'jock' itch.

Special senses
Blurred vision; tinnitus.

Digestive system
Having a rumbling tummy; feeling starving when you have not eaten for a few hours.

Mental/psychological symptoms
An inability to think clearly or find words; feeling spaced out or dizzy; depression; lack of confidence; irritability; tearfulness. Only feeling normal when you have consumed and/or being addicted to sugar, carbohydrate, chocolate, caffeine or alcohol. Losing control and consuming large quantities of the above.

Miscellaneous
Waking in the early hours of the morning as blood sugar levels fall and adrenaline levels surge; night sweats; feeling weak, faint, shaky or unable to concentrate when you have not eaten for a few hours.

Please refer to figure 11 for the signs and symptoms of poor pancreatic function or insulin resistance. The pancreas can be affected by toxic metals and microbes in the same way as the other endocrine organs and may be particularly vulnerable to electromagnetic radiation and 'dirty' electricity. The pancreas has a high requirement for chromium and deficiency of this mineral may lead to pancreatic malfunction. The use of baby formula may also be implicated in initiating autoimmune disease of the pancreas and wheat lectins are known to mimic insulin and may further confound the issue.

The specific dietary requirements for addressing blood sugar control are discussed in chapter 14. If you are diabetic please monitor your blood glucose closely throughout detoxification and inform the appropriate health care practitioner of any changes.

The Emotional Meaning of Pancreatic Dysfunction

On an emotional level, the pancreas relates to issues of parenthood, specifically to the loss of a child through miscarriage, abortion, death, adoption or separation and also to issues of being separated from your mother. The loss of a child may refer to an early miscarriage that could have passed unnoticed or was thought to be a late, heavy period (50 per cent of pregnancies are thought to end in this way). Alternatively, the majority of pregnancies (estimated at 70 per cent) start out as twins, with one foetus being sacrificed in order to bring the other to term. This means that the parents involved would not necessarily be consciously aware of their loss although it will impact them on a biological and/or spiritual level. This also applies to men and can set up grossly dysfunctional eating patterns with a lot of comfort eating and excessive weight gain. For example, some women's lifelong problems with food may be related to a miscarriage or stillbirth in their youth. The uterus can go into a kind of grief (even if you think that you have come to terms with whatever happened – or that it was a long time ago) and can start to grow fibroids or similar in a frustrated attempt to grow something. Problems with the pancreas also relate generally to a feeling that, for you, life is not sweet and a feeling of hopelessness and anxiety about the future.

Disorders of the Ovaries and Testes

The testes in men are invariably involved in FRS and this can cause impotence, loss of libido and infertility. In women the ovaries are affected causing an irregular menstrual cycle, prolonged or irregular bleeding, excessively painful periods, infertility, PMS, loss of libido, miscarriage and breast tenderness.

There is a complex relationship between the female sex hormone, oestrogen, and mercury which is both oestrogenic (oestrogen-loving) and an oestrogen mimic (a xeno-oestrogen). Oestrogen encourages the deposition of fat and breast growth in women and causes feminization and gynaecomastia (or 'man-boobs') in men, whereas the other major female sex hormone, progesterone, promotes the relaxation of smooth muscle and a deficiency can cause the kind of spasms involved in IBS and asthma. Pre-menopausal and pregnant women have enhanced liver detoxification phase 1 activity compared to men or post-menopausal women and this may partially explain the toxic build-up of metabolites and the disproportionate number of female FRS sufferers. An inability to methylate oestrogens in the liver due to mercury toxicity may also be implicated in the development of autoimmune disease and may explain the predominance of these disorders in women. Finally, excess circulating oestrogen also promotes the overgrowth of fungi such as Candida.

The Emotional Meaning of Gonadal Dysfunction

Emotional issues that relate to dysfunction of the reproductive organs include any regrets, stubbornness, jealousy and sexual tension.

Master Gland Dysfunction

The controlling glands deep in the brain are the pineal (which regulates sleep/wake cycles), the hypothalamus (which is a bundle of nerve tissue and sensors) and the pituitary gland (that acts as a store of hormones). The hypothalamus is intimately involved in all FRS and it may ultimately be these controlling glands that are responsible for the endocrine problems witnessed in FRS. The pituitary gland is also vulnerable to physical trauma, hanging as it does by a stalk from the base of the brain. Any accidents serious enough to have rendered someone temporarily unconscious at any time may have sustained unrecognized damage to this gland. In order to address these complex issues, you definitely need to recruit someone experienced and knowledgeable in this field.

Chapter 11

Causative Emotional Issues

Medicine is only palliative, for back of disease lies the cause, and this no drug can reach.

Dr Weir Mitchel

Amateur psychologists can never quite decide whether FRS is the end result of a perfectionistic, driven personality ('yuppie flu') or whether sufferers are work-shy, self-absorbed hypochondriacs. The ultimate irony is that the typical FRS sufferer is someone who has driven themselves to exhaustion and then when they finally and inevitably collapse, they are accused of laziness!

The fact is that emotional and spiritual issues are ultimately *the cause of all disease* and FRS is no exception. In fact, the Center for Disease Control (CDC) states that 85 per cent of all disease is partially or wholly emotional – and yet these issues are only just starting to be addressed by allopathic medicine. The truth is that you cannot heal your body without healing your psyche since they are interrelated and holographic aspects of the self. This means addressing the underlying emotional and/or spiritual issues that caused you to become so ill in the first place in order to prevent a recurrence of this or some other dread disease. Emotions have played a large part in initiating and perpetuating your FRS and the more willing you are to examine *everything*, the more likely you are to get well. The goal of the emotional aspects of treatment is to help you to understand and come to terms with unresolved issues and in so doing allow stored toxins to be released and excreted.

The Subconscious

The subconscious is vast and has many millions of times the computing speed of the conscious mind; it has stored a complete and accurate record of every event in your life outside of the concept of time. Conscious memory begins with the acquisition of language and although memories prior to this are recorded they cannot usually be accessed. It is now known that children are in a hypnagogic state until they are about seven years old, during which time they have no discrimination. During these formative years they download the 'software programme' unconsciously given to them primarily by their parents into their subconscious mind. The individual then operates out of this programme which effectively runs their life on 'autopilot' the vast majority of the time, with the conscious mind often only intervening when things have gone 'wrong'. Addressing the conscious mind (as in conventional psychotherapy and psychiatry) is very time-consuming and has not proven to be very successful in effecting change – most probably because the conscious mind literally *was not present* most of the time and is almost certainly not the cause of the 'problem'. You may wonder why you never have enough money, attract the wrong sort of partner or you became so ill – and the answer is invariably to be found in your subconscious mind which knows exactly what the causative issues are. Individuals also see themselves through this downloaded programme so no matter how little factual basis there is for the belief, if they were told they were ugly, stupid or worthless then they subconsciously attract behaviour throughout life that validates this belief and further traumatizes them.

> **Give me a child until he is seven and I will give you the man.**
>
> **Jesuit motto**

Trauma

We are currently experiencing an epidemic of chronic disease, which may have many causes (addressed elsewhere in this book); however, repeated trauma is a prime candidate. One study showed a direct correlation between the number of minor adverse life events and major causes of death, addiction, substance abuse and mental illness. A trauma is defined as a life stress that occurs in a state of helplessness and all of us are thought to have been traumatized in some way – and often repeatedly. In fact, trauma may begin in the womb and be compounded by our experience of a difficult birth which may have burned a deep memory of entry into this world as being terrifying. Breastfeeding is also now thought to be very important not only for the health benefits, but because the mother produces oxytocin which aids bonding. This hormone also promotes the proper development of the autonomic nervous system and the emotional brain required to produce a physically and emotionally resilient adult. This early empathic care is thought to be very important, so having a mother who suffered post-natal depression, mental illness or who was neglectful has a profound and lasting effect on the developing child. The once popular practices of letting babies cry and of keeping them from their mothers to allow the mothers to rest, may have been experienced as both terror and abandonment by the baby who may have been deeply traumatized by these procedures.

Thereafter there is the usual conflict with siblings, being unfairly punished at some stage, having a loved relative or friend die and being bullied. For many, though, the default setting was that they were happy and not unduly stressed for most of their childhood. However, it is estimated that at least one quarter of children have been sexually, physically or emotionally abused in homes where there was overt dysfunction. Many of these children may have been so overwhelmed by painful and powerful emotions early in life that they effectively unconsciously decided that living inside their heads was preferable to living inside their bodies and FRS may be the ultimate consequence of this decision. Alternatively, there may be some form of covert dysfunction within the family where problems were not acknowledged, but there were all sorts of tensions beneath the surface. This environment can create chronic social stress in the one place that should be a 'safe' refuge from the outside world.

A Child's Eye View

What is important to understand is how you would have experienced events as a child and not how you think about them now from the perspective of adulthood. The most threatening thing that can happen to a child is the perceived threat of desertion which usually means death in the animal kingdom. As a child you are vulnerable and totally dependent on the grown-ups in your world and even your mother being late to pick you up from school may have led to strong feelings of fear and abandonment. Also, no matter how much you may love them now, most people who have younger siblings probably experienced their introduction to the family with jealousy and as a rejection and a threat. After all, witnessing your parents lavishing loving attention on the new arrival must be galling unless handled very sensitively. Children also often perceive themselves as being to blame for adult problems and many may have internalized a programme that said that they had to be perfect in order to be loved. Nothing can wear someone out quite like setting the bar so high for every activity that it is impossible for themselves and others to reach the standards that they have set and yet equally impossible to request help. If this is you, it is time to accept that you are not perfect because no one is, and that being perfect does not actually make you loveable or win you any friends. You are fine just as you are.

How Trauma Impacts Health

One mechanism as to how historic emotions can permanently affect health was developed by the neurobiologist and medical doctor, Dietrich Klinghardt. This involves the organs of detoxification being temporarily compromised by trauma, enabling toxins – and particularly neurotoxins like mercury – to be absorbed into the nerve endings of the autonomic nervous system. These toxins enter under the auspices of the emotional right brain and relentlessly track up the nerves, progressively compromising function of the affected organs and eventually concentrating in the central nervous system. The manner in which this happens has long been acknowledged by Traditional Chinese Medicine with, for example, toxins accumulating in the liver in response to anger or resentment, in the gall bladder due to rage, in the kidneys due to fear, and in the large intestine due to guilt. The permeability of the blood–brain barrier also increases with stress, making the individual more vulnerable to toxicity of the central nervous system and hypothalamus at these times. In this manner, early life trauma can produce grave symptoms decades later. After all, those with essentially happy childhoods have been exposed to many of the same toxins as those with traumatic childhoods, but have emerged at least seemingly unscathed as a result of their ability to detoxify efficiently. There are also several other proposed mechanisms by which early life trauma can have a lasting effect on your health and well-being. It can certainly prove challenging not only to identify and acknowledge, but to release these traumatic events, however, this process is a very necessary part of your healing.

> Our nervous system isn't just a fiction, it's part of our physical body, and our soul exists in space and is inside us, like teeth in our mouth. It can't be forever violated with impunity.
>
> **Boris Pasternak**

Post-Traumatic Stress

Sometimes you can be morbidly aware of the causative issue because the memories haunt you and these events often occurred later in childhood. Alternatively, some events are deemed so traumatic that the psyche edits the memory from conscious awareness, burying it in the subconscious mind, and this is thought to occur more often with early life trauma. Memory repression often occurs with a car accident, for instance, and whilst this mechanism may aid short-term survival and prevent flashbacks, these repressed memories 'leak' into the conscious mind and must find expression in some form – often including chronic ill health. In this way, some of the events that may be having a significant effect upon your health are memories that have been completely repressed.

Sexual Abuse

Sexual abuse is by no means unusual, but may not always be consciously remembered, and although little boys are sometimes the victims, sexual abuse of girls is more common. The perpetrator is much more likely to have been a family member or a trusted friend than the predatory stranger that most parents fear. As an adult, leakage of these repressed memories occurs in repetitive nightmares, troubling and intrusive thoughts, body sensations and body 'memories', feelings about sexual contact, the perpetrator or the environment in which the abuse occurred, and sexual responsiveness. All of which may serve as clues to indicate a repressed memory of abuse. The most profound traumas have often been inflicted by a loved caregiver, meaning that the child can also become terribly conflicted. This may result in depression as a result of repressing the anger and rage felt and in chronically low self-esteem and self-loathing as a result of internalizing feelings of disgust and worthlessness. All of this creates a toxic cauldron of suppressed powerful emotions which may ultimately give rise to serious or chronic ill health. Sadly, the abused individual often takes this subconscious emotional template forward in their life and attracts further abuse as an adult. Many women who subsequently become involved in violent relationships are believed to have experienced abuse of some kind as a child. Likewise, the majority of abusers are thought to have themselves experienced abuse at the hands of a loved one – whether they consciously remember it or not. Sex hormones are also known to be produced precociously during sexual abuse and this may initiate endocrine dysfunction. This understanding brings a whole new meaning to the term a 'victim' of FRS.

> A bodily disease may be but a symptom of some ailment in the spiritual past.
>
> **Nathaniel Hawthorne**

You and Your Shadow

We all have a 'shadow side' to our personality and the more likely you are to deny it, the more seriously in trouble you are. This is the side of us that we don't own or acknowledge and that we definitely do not present to the world – but actually it is just the unknown. In order to get really and truly well you have to resolve to stop running from your shadow and turn and face it down once and for all. This is not an easy task and will require a great deal of courage. This process has probably been enshrined in the mythical journey of a hero fighting dragons and demons when entering the underworld in some form. Your shadow is responsible for the less-than-kind feelings you sometimes harbour and for the occasions on which you think, 'Why did I do/say that?' Your shadow can and will sabotage your best conscious efforts. Those who have confronted their shadow and have come out on the other side of this experience, have a palpable quality about them. My guess is that Nelson Mandela achieved this while incarcerated.

Intergenerational Dynamics

Sometimes, you may also need to examine the wider family dynamic, because people can unknowingly take on 'emotional baggage' that does not belong to them but has been passed down to them from a previous generation. There may be a family member within the last two generations who has been excluded or rejected by the family. This may be a baby that died that no one ever speaks of, someone who was mentally ill or someone who is perceived to have been disgraced in some way. These historic events within the family are like boulders upstream in a river that can create turbulence downstream – possibly in your life. It is thought that, probably at a soul level, there are no such things as secrets within a family and that all members know everything – although they may not be consciously aware that they know. In this way the fact that your father had a series of affairs or that your mother was actually in love with someone other than your father set up family dynamics that are toxic, stressful and hard to identify.

The Affected Chakras

Of the seven main energy centres or chakras, it is the three lower chakras which relate to the physical world and your formative experiences of it that are most commonly affected in FRS. The organs that are most impacted will give you clues as to what the causative emotional issue(s) might be.

- The base chakra (near the coccyx) relates to issues of 'home', grounding and feeling connected to your body. The organs affected by base chakra issues are the adrenal glands, kidneys, bladder, colon, legs and spine.
- The sacral chakra (mid-belly) relates to feelings in general, one-to-one relationships, sexuality and issues around finance and security in particular.

These issues tend to manifest in problems with the reproductive organs and spleen/immune system.
- The solar plexus chakra (upper abdomen) relates to your feelings about yourself, your self-esteem and assertiveness. The organs affected are the pancreas, stomach, liver, gall bladder and sympathetic nervous system.

What Your Body Is Trying to Tell You

Science alone can't cure or help people. Illness is individual. Each person is unique, and diseases are connected to their hearts.

Dr Shigeaki Hinohara

The body is always helpfully trying to represent in physical form the spiritual and emotional issues that you most need to address. For instance, the body parts all have associated meanings, with the back being widely regarded as representing emotional or financial support; the shoulders our ability to bear burdens; the legs our capacity to move forwards and the hands our potential to handle the issues of life. The bowels relate to releasing the past; the liver to anger; stiff muscles to a lack of flexibility and stiff joints to rigid attitudes. The particular conditions also have associated meanings, with asthma relating to feelings of being smothered; deafness to not wanting to hear; cystitis to being 'pissed off'; incontinence to letting go; the presence of parasites to some kind of parasitic energy relationship (usually with someone close); depression to repressed anger. Ask to be shown what your body is metaphorically trying to represent for you. You can often see the truth of other people's disorders, but your own may be invisible to you because these conditions often represent aspects of yourself that you reject and you may need to ask a trusted friend who can perhaps see you more objectively. For further information on this subject, you may want to read the work of Louise Hay which details the body parts and disorders and their associated meanings.

You may find that many of your symptoms are on one side of your body and this too can give you an indication of their provenance. The right-hand side of the body relates to the male both within you and to your relationship with specific men, most probably a father or father figure. The left-hand side of your body relates to your feminine aspect and your relationship with women, most probably your mother.

Finally, consider the possibility that having a fatigue-related syndrome itself can also be an unconscious way of attention seeking. Some of these patterns may have been set up a long time ago and obviously they are deeply unwelcome now. Were you somewhat neglected as a child? Perhaps you have been disappointed by your life in other ways and your disease gives you a perverse power? Honestly confront what may be true.

Dissociation

> **Diseases of the soul are more dangerous and more numerous than those of the body.**
>
> **Cicero**

You are an immortal soul having a mortal human experience and your physical body is an instrument or vehicle with which you can experience this reality. When severe trauma is experienced, the part of the soul carrying the trauma can dissociate permanently outside of time and space. This is a survival mechanism that enables you to keep going and the soul returns at night, which is why you may have dreams reliving the traumatic event. This is a common response to traumas including birth trauma, being abused or neglected, miscarriage or abortion, a near death experience, car accidents, divorce or betrayal and wartime experiences. It is a primary cause of premature death and serious illness. Classic signs of dissociation are blocked memory – either of an event, a person, a house or an age – and that the person becomes emotionally remote, chronically negative and feels apathetic, listless, despairing or becomes addicted to a substance or substances. If you feel that you were *never the same again* after some traumatic life event and you can identify with the above signs, then it might be worth seeking out a spiritual or shamanic healer experienced in soul retrieval.

Part 2

The Solutions

Health is a state of complete physical, mental and social well-being, and not merely the absence of disease or infirmity.

World Health Organization, 1948

I know God will not give me anything I can't handle. I just wish that He didn't trust me so much.

Mother Teresa

Chapter 12

The FRS Natural Recovery Plan

Never, no never, did Nature say one thing and
Wisdom say another.

Edmund Burke

As you probably appreciate by now, you are primarily suffering from an iatrogenic disease caused by an extremely potent neurotoxin and, secondarily, the microbes and their biotoxins that have prospered in its presence. Part 1 addressed the background information that you need to understand in order to put in place the solutions offered in Part 2 of this book. Please refer to figure 12, which shows the processes of toxification and the routes of detoxification.

It may help you to think of the body as a house where new goods are constantly

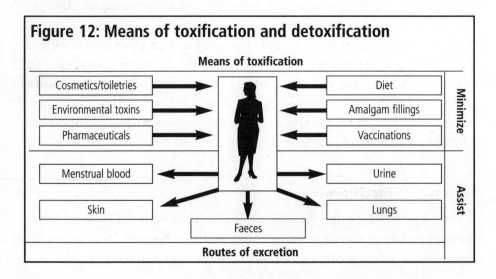

Figure 12: Means of toxification and detoxification

Means of toxification

Cosmetics/toiletries	Diet
Environmental toxins	Amalgam fillings
Pharmaceuticals	Vaccinations

Minimize

Menstrual blood	Urine
Skin	Lungs
	Faeces

Assist

Routes of excretion

being brought in through the front door, and where the solid refuse is generally taken out through the back door and collected and the sewage system carries away waste liquids. If these disposal mechanisms are not working properly for whatever reason, then the incoming stuff starts backing up within the house. Now, you may choose to fill the spare bedroom and cupboard space before you start stacking belongings up in the living room, but you need to try and keep the hallways negotiable. Over time it becomes progressively harder to function and decomposing possessions might start to create real problems in some locations.

The equivalent of our 'modern' medical answer to this dilemma is to have specially trained people treat the house with sophisticated chemicals or demolish the offending room! The less high tech, but nonetheless effective approach is to minimize and monitor the amount of incoming material and to re-establish the mechanisms for refuse and sewage disposal and ensure that they are maintained. Then you need to start clearing out the backlog in the hallways and on the stairs before pulling more rubbish out of the other rooms. In Part 2 we are going to examine this holistic approach to optimizing the systems that already exist and which you can largely manage yourself.

If it's complex – it's from ego.

Spiritual principle

You are going to need to take simultaneous action in several different arenas of your life in order to recover and the following chapters address these subjects as shown in figure 13. What counts is not getting things perfect, but taking regular small steps on all fronts and then sustaining the changes over time. This does not all have to happen overnight, however, try to resist the gravitational pull back towards the habits and choices that made you sick in the first place. You may want to draw up an action plan as you read through the following chapters and then decide specifically what you are going to do. Bear in mind also that all disease shares a common root so your efforts will also help to prevent some of the more horrendous diseases of old age. If you ever find that progress is slow or that you are relapsing, take stock and re-institute the basics. Better yet, do everything you know you need to do to get well all of the time.

Finding a Practitioner

It is strongly recommended that you try and locate a practitioner versed in the treatment of metal toxicity to guide your treatment. They will be able to tailor treatment to your specific requirements and both monitor your progress and change

Figure 13: The six elements of the FRS natural recovery plan

1.	Chapter 13	**Cleaning up your environment**
2.	Chapter 14	**Eating a nutritious diet**
3.	Chapter 15	**Sorting out emotional issues**
4.	Chapter 16	**Developing a lifestyle that supports healing**
5.	Chapter 17	**Taking supplements**
6.	Chapter 18	**Possible revision of dental work**

your supplementation dynamically as your needs change throughout treatment. In the long run this will save you both time and money as they can more efficiently oversee your recovery and can also provide the reassurance you may need on occasions. Many clients initially present with bags of 30 or more supplements that they are taking that they had read might help. The problem with this approach is that it is very expensive and may not be very helpful. First, taking anything that the body does not actually require is a waste of money, as these products will either be eliminated using the usual channels or stored. Secondly, every supplement taken has to be detoxified by the liver and this is giving an already struggling organ more work to do. This approach can actually be counterproductive too because some nutrients need to be taken separately from others whilst some are best taken in combination with other supplements – a practitioner should be well versed in such matters. Last, but not least, there is the very real and serious danger of mobilizing toxins out of storage without adequately supporting the organs of excretion first. This can lead to *retoxification*, whereby toxins that have been stowed away over a period of years in relatively safe storage in structures such as the joints and muscles are mobilized and re-deposited in more vulnerable body compartments such as the brain or heart.

Some doctors have a special interest in the treatment of metal toxicity and may offer detoxification using intravenous chelating agents and this may help to expedite the detoxification process. This approach may, however, prove quite expensive and you should bear in mind that for every expensive laboratory test or procedure you could, for instance, have taken a lot of supplements or had a course of colonics.

Chapter 13

Reducing Toxin Exposure

> The consideration of man's body has not changed to meet the new condition of this artificial environment that has replaced his natural one. The result of this … perpetual discord is a general deterioration of man's body, the symptoms of which are termed disease.
>
> **Professor Hilton Hotema**

In this chapter we examine the different actions that you need to take in order to substantially reduce your future exposure to environmental toxins and look at some of the chief culprits in more detail.

Quit Smoking

It is not for nothing that smoking-related illnesses will prematurely kill half of all people who smoke and that smokers often look so much older than their years. Cigarettes contain at least 400 toxins which become suspended in an aerosol, maximizing absorption, and are heated so that they are at their most destructive during smoking. In fact, every puff of smoke is estimated to contain *over a trillion reactive oxygen species* which cause massive oxidative damage throughout the body. Smoking is recognized to prolong the healing process and greatly increase complications after surgery, for instance, and so is working against all your best efforts in other arenas to recover. If you smoke and suffer with FRS then quitting is the single most important action you can take to preserve and reclaim your health. If someone else in your household smokes then try to get them to agree to smoke in another room or outside.

Cosmetics and Toiletries

It is estimated that the average woman applies over 200 chemicals to her skin each day and that up to 70 per cent of these are absorbed and thus have to be detoxified and then either excreted or stored. In fact, up to 2kg (4.4lb) of toxins are believed to be assimilated in this way each year. Somewhat remarkably, although new ingredients are required to be tested for safety, the vast majority of constituents that have traditionally been used are *assumed to be safe* although this has never been demonstrated. There is particular concern about three chemicals that are commonly used in body care products and which are all known toxins. The first of these is propylene glycol which is used to emulsify components in moisturizers, cosmetics and other products. Second is sodium lauryl sulphate which is used as a foaming agent in shampoos, toothpastes, body washes and bubble baths. Third are phthalates which are used as a solvent and plasticizer in cosmetics, perfumes and nail polish. There are now good selections of reasonably priced, pleasant, natural organic toiletries and cosmetics available in health food shops and over the Internet such as Dr Hauschka, Jurlique and Weleda. Some new powdered mineral cosmetics are currently becoming available that do not use many of the toxic ingredients associated with other products. It is important to scrutinize labels, because any product that is natural and organic will be proud to let you know, but labelling generally can be deceptive. Try to avoid using some products altogether where possible such as hairspray, body sprays, talcum powder, mouthwashes and perfume.

> **Vitality and beauty are gifts of Nature for those who live according to its laws.**
>
> **Leonardo Da Vinci**

Antiperspirants

Nearly all antiperspirants contain aluminium (unless specifically labelled otherwise) and the thin, hot, moist skin of your underarms easily absorbs this. There is particular concern about women using these products which are thought to compromise lymphatic drainage of the breasts. There are now reasonably priced aluminium-free alternatives available. You should avoid using feminine hygiene or body sprays for similar reasons.

Household Chemicals

Most indoor environments are much more toxic than even fairly polluted outdoor environments, with measurements of some pollutants being up to *a hundred times higher* in indoor air. For this reason and because you spend so much time there, it is important to clean up your home environment as much as possible. The average home is estimated to store more than 60 toxic products, so have a clear out and throw away any unused cans of paint or the various other chemicals used for cleaning paths and preserving wood. Certainly do not store these products in the house or in a garage attached to the house. Generally, try to avoid using chemicals in the garden, such as lawn treatments and patio cleaners, and also eliminate products that you don't have to use like air fresheners, fabric softeners and antibacterial sprays. Keep your house clean, but you should not need to use lots of chemicals and, remember, if you can smell it – your body has to detoxify it. You can make your own cleaning products or buy eco-products either over the Internet, in the supermarket or at health food shops.

If your carpet has seen better days, arrange to have it professionally cleaned using a chemical-free process and then invest in a good-quality vacuum cleaner (one approved for use for asthmatics) and use it to clean thoroughly every week, including soft furnishings. Have everyone change into slippers when they come indoors so that they do not bring parasite eggs in on the soles of their shoes and then walk them into the carpets.

If having building work done, be aware that house fumigation and timber treatment fumes can persist for years afterwards, as can the flame retardants that are used to treat carpets, curtains and soft furnishings. Most gloss paints contain volatile organic compounds (VOC) derived from petrochemicals and these can produce protracted flu-like symptoms. Obviously the person doing the painting has high levels of exposure at the time of the application, however those who then live or sleep in the room have a continuous low level of exposure for many months afterwards. Many manufacturers are now introducing low-fume paints, which might be slightly better, whilst other companies produce environmentally friendly paints or water-based paints for use on metal and wood. Also, when using any chemical products ensure that if the instructions include the advice to 'ensure adequate ventilation' or to wear protective gloves or a mask that you do just that.

Other sources of fumes include low-level leaks from either the gas mains supply, the central heating system or gas appliances. Traffic pollution is probably unavoidable if you live on a busy main road, but if you have a garage attached to the house consider sealing the door and using another entrance. Avoid dry cleaning items when possible and if you do, remove the bag and leave the clothes in a ventilated area. Open windows on a regular basis and both deionizers and air conditioners may help if you suffer from respiratory allergies.

Exposure at Work

If you are exposed to chemicals at work and think that your job may be contributing to your ill health, then you need to consider other alternatives or ask for protective clothing and equipment if appropriate. If you are not even sure what risks you might be exposed to ask to see the health and safety risk assessment. At the very least, make sure that your diet is optimal and take some professional advice about supplementing so that you can detoxify the chemicals to which you are routinely exposed.

Inhalant Allergies

Many FRS sufferers have multiple allergies and these *will slowly subside* as you detoxify. In the interim, techniques such as Nambudripad's Allergy Elimination Techniques (otherwise known as NAET), homeopathic desensitization, kinesiology and various energy-tapping techniques may provide relief of symptoms (see also supplement suggestions in figure 34).

Environmental Stresses
Geopathic Stress

If you suspect that geopathic or underground water stress (as discussed in chapter 6) may be a causative issue in your FRS, you could try rearranging key pieces of furniture or using a different room for your bedroom or office. Some devices are also available which claim to negate the effect, however, ideally you would recruit a 'house healer' or dowser who specializes in treating geopathic stress.

Electromagnetic Stress

If you think that electromagnetic stress might be contributing to your FRS, then consider the following:

- Remove or unplug *all* electrical equipment in the bedroom, especially from around the *head of the bed* where the electromagnetic field can detrimentally affect your brain for 8 hours a day. Metal deposits within the body are also thought to act as antennae, further sensitizing the metal-toxic individual to electromagnetic fields. Get a battery alarm clock, remove electric blankets, do not sleep in a metal frame bed and do not leave a mobile phone switched on next to the bed.

- Mattresses containing metal springs can be tested for electromagnetic emissions by moving a fluid-filled compass over the surface of the bed. Replacement with a foam mattress may be necessary.
- You can purchase various protective devices such as a screen for your computer monitor or a new low-radiation computer screen and chips for the back of your mobile phone. Avoid wireless computers and other wireless systems wherever possible and certainly turn Wi-Fi systems off when not in use.
- There are various plug-in devices available for protecting the home or workspace and items that can be worn or carried to protect the individual.
- Ideally, don't microwave and certainly don't stand next to the microwave while it is on.
- Use a landline telephone with a cable whenever possible, rather than a cordless phone. If you carry a mobile phone, turn it off when not in use and don't always keep it in the same pocket or carry it in your bag on the same side of your body. The new generation of video-imaging mobile phones uses a stronger signal than the previous generation, so don't upgrade unless necessary.
- It is also possible to rent an electromagnetic pollution meter or to get someone to assess your home or workspace for a fee.

Chapter 14

The FRS Diet

The doctor of the future will no longer treat the human frame with drugs, but rather will cure and prevent disease with nutrition.

Thomas Edison

The developed world is facing a tsunami of chronic and degenerative illnesses largely caused by diet. Whereas a normal breakfast in Japan or Thailand might be fish and rice, in the developed world it is currently more likely to be some combination of sweetened and refined wheat and dairy products. These culturally acquired norms are the result of learned preferences and countless generations of human intervention in animal husbandry and crop cultivation. For instance, the wheat that we now eat bears little relationship to the wheat our ancestors would have recognized a thousand years ago and the gluten molecule is now twice the length it was then and in the process has become less digestible. The advent of dairy farming also meant that milk that had formerly come from sheep or goats primarily started to come from cows. Cow's milk has a longer casein molecule than that of sheep or goats and the recent introduction of pasteurization and low-fat milks all conspire to make it harder to digest. Recognize that what is accepted as 'normal' may not be good or even desirable. Your diet is going to play a key role in aiding detoxification and in repairing and rebuilding damaged tissue. Your nutritional status is dependent on the food that you eat and on the efficiency of your digestion and absorption processes. You may need to seriously upgrade your ideas about nutrition and what a desirable diet should be in order to recover from FRS.

Where to Begin

In order to control what is in your food you are going to need to cook everything from scratch using organic ingredients wherever possible. Although this can be hard work, it is the most worthwhile investment you can make in your own health – and that of your family. The 'French paradox' refers to the unusually high consumption of meat, dairy produce and alcohol in France and yet very low levels of heart disease and obesity. This finding may relate more to the fact that they buy local, fresh produce and take pride in cooking rather than relying on the ready meals that have become common in other countries. Whilst supermarket fruit and vegetables may look fresh, they have often been sprayed with fertilizers and pesticides, harvested 'green', kept in a modified atmosphere for months and then ripened using ethylene gas. Try to buy local produce, arrange for delivery of an organic box scheme, or better yet – grow your own. Buy organic meat where possible to avoid the pesticides, antibiotics, growth hormones and vaccines used in rearing regular meat. Venison, lamb, pheasant or duck can be good options because they are less likely to have been subject to these farming methods. Try and purchase food and drinks in glass containers or bottles rather than in cans as both the metal and the chemical used to treat it (Bisphenol A) are toxic and leach into the product. Try to buy as few foods as possible with labels on, and if you do, examine the label carefully and know that it probably does not tell the whole story. Any foods that have a long shelf-life are 'dead' foods and should be kept to a minimum. This diet can make eating away from home difficult and the key is to plan ahead by, for instance, taking a thermos of soup into work and when eating out to choose the simplest foods such as fish or meat with salad or vegetables. The diet that all FRS sufferers need to follow is effectively a modern take on the Stone Age diet that our ancestors ate for many millennia before the advent of agriculture, and meal suggestions are shown in figure 14.

Figure 14: FRS meal suggestions

Meal	Options
Breakfast	Oatmeal or rice porridge; sugar-free or homemade muesli (gluten-free if necessary); unsweetened oat cereals; boiled egg and oatcakes; fruit; scrambled eggs with smoked salmon; bacon, tomatoes and sautéed potatoes; brown rice kedgeree; buckwheat pancakes and berries; gluten-free cereal and rice milk.
Lunch	Meat, fish and/or vegetable soups; salads with chicken, fish or meat; rice salad; leftovers like casserole; sushi; a baked potato with prawns (no mayonnaise), tuna or homemade chilli; oatcakes with homemade fish paté or cold meat; fruit or fruit salad.
Evening meal	Meat, poultry or fish with vegetables and homemade sauce or gravy; spelt or rice pasta with homemade sauce; chicken, prawn or meat stir-fry with rice or rice noodles; risotto; homemade curry with rice; casserole or stew and potatoes.

Below we examine the 'good' foods that need to be included in your diet as much as possible to support your recovery, the 'bad' foods that should be avoided as much as possible and finally, the 'ugly' foods that should be excluded entirely.

The 'Good' Foods

Let food be thy medicine, and let thy medicine be food.

Hippocrates

Fibre

It is critical that you establish and maintain regular bowel movements – not only for the duration of the detoxification, but for the rest of your days. Eating a healthy diet of fibrous whole foods will bulk out the stool and will prevent re-absorption into the body of the bile in which the toxins are being excreted. Soluble fibre is found in foods such as oats, dried beans and apples and insoluble fibre is found in whole grains, nuts, seeds, fruits and vegetables. Aim to include at least five portions of fruit or vegetables a day and try to eat a variety of colours as the pigments are antioxidants (proanthocyanidins) with different actions. Cook vegetables as little as possible using steaming or stir-frying and aim to eat at least some food raw every day either as crudités, fruit or as a salad. Include a reasonable amount of carbohydrates in as unrefined a state as is possible, such as wholegrain rice, potato, porridge oats and oatcakes (if tolerated), lentils, beans and chickpeas. The exceptions to this rule may be those with seriously compromised digestive systems, but even so you can still include plenty of fibre in hearty vegetable soups without the abrasive effect of some whole grains.

Protein

It is now recognized that detoxification is an entirely nutrient-dependent process. If your liver does not have all the nutrients required to detoxify a substance, then these toxins will be temporarily stored until such time as the nutrients become available. Of course, for many the appropriate nutrients never do become available – or at least not in sufficient quantities – and so the inexorable descent into toxicity and illness begins unheralded. Two of the six phase II liver detoxification pathways that are particularly affected by mercury toxicity are the methylation and sulphation pathways. The methylation pathway is responsible for metabolizing fats, DNA and oestrogen; and the sulphation pathway for processing neurotransmitters, thyroid and steroid hormones, toxins from bowel flora and other substances such as paracetamol (acetominophen).

These pathways derive the methyl and sulphur groups required for conjugation primarily from methionine which is an amino acid largely found in meat and fish. So in order to be able to detoxify metals and also to provide the proteins required to repair and renew the extensive tissue damage associated with FRS you need to be eating high-quality animal protein at least twice, and ideally three times a day. A portion of protein is approximately the size of a pack of playing cards and acceptable high-quality animal proteins include eggs, cheese, meat or fish.

It is simply not possible to detoxify metals effectively on a vegan diet (there is relatively little methionine in beans and nuts) and the likelihood of you getting better if you don't introduce some animal source protein is negligible. If you are vegan and are determined to stay that way, then the addition of a high-quality protein drink at mealtimes or supplementing L-carnitine may help. If you are a lacto-vegetarian, make sure that you are eating properly balanced, nutritious meals and include eggs and cheese (if you are not intolerant) in your diet along with all the other sources of protein, and consider including some fish. Vegetarian or not, supplementing a cow or goat whey-based protein drink can provide valuable support for detoxification. Alternatively, now that you are seriously ill, you might want to reconsider your stance on consuming animal protein. It is really only in the last century or so that some have chosen on ethical or health grounds to exclude all animal products, but historically we have evolved to eat at least small amounts of animal protein. A lot of vegetarians also rely heavily on wheat and dairy as dietary staples – which are the two main food allergens. Whilst some peoples have successfully managed vegetarianism over centuries, they tend to have different blood types and typically live in hot, sunny climates that for all their privations do not present the toxic challenge encountered by many in developed countries.

'Good' Fats

In the recent hysteria over fats, people have reduced their intake of 'good' fats along with the 'bad' fats found in processed foods and meats as shown in figure 15. The 'good' fats include two polyunsaturated fats the body cannot make which are referred to as essential fatty acids (EFA). These EFAs act as starting points for the synthesis of many essential fats within the body and are required for processes such as energy production, oxygen transport, proper immune function and the synthesis of hormones. One family of EFAs is known as omega 3 oils and these are found mostly in fish, and the other is known as omega 6 oils and these are found in meat, and nuts and seeds and their oils.

Figure 15: Fats and their properties

Oil		Source
Good oils Monounsaturated		Avocado; nuts and their oils; olives and olive oil
Polyunsaturated fats – Omega 3		Dark oily fish and some cold water fish; seeds and their oils; dark green leafy vegetables; soybeans; O3 oils; O3 eggs; O3 supplemented milk
	Omega 6	Meat; poultry; dairy; eggs; wheatgerm; nuts and seeds and their oils; soybean and its products
Saturated fats		Coconut and its oils are regarded as 'good' saturated fats
Bad oils Saturated		Red meat; butter; cheese; cream; lard; coconut; vegetable shortening
Hydrogenated and trans-fats		Margarine; manufactured food; potato chips; shortening; chocolate; ice cream; baked goods

Almost everyone (unless they are already supplementing) is deficient in omega 3 oils, mostly due to food processing and the fact that oily fish consumption has dropped by 80 per cent in recent years as the population switched from a standard kipper breakfast to cereals. These omega 3 oils comprise up to *three-quarters* of the dry weight of the brain and deficiency makes the nervous system vulnerable to the metallic mercury vapour from amalgam fillings and to depression. Omega 3 oils and the omega 6 oils from safflower and sunflower oil are also converted within the body into prostaglandins which are a subgroup of eicosanoids which are locally acting hormones that reduce inflammation and control immunity. Figure 16 shows the relationship of the various omega 3 oils, of which eicosapentanoic acid (EPA) is the most beneficial to the nervous system and is converted relatively poorly from vegetable source alpha linolenic acid (ALA). Do not worry at all about good fats making you fat – they simply don't. In fact, quite the opposite, with good fats aiding energy production and fat-burning. Seeds are rich sources of the good oils, so snack on them whenever possible, sprinkle whole onto cereal or salad or grind them in a coffee grinder before use to make them more digestible if your digestion is compromised. Keep seeds in the refrigerator and use before the specified date.

A good-quality olive oil is ideal for general use in cooking and dressings, but it should be stored in a dark glass bottle in the refrigerator and not allowed to smoke or be re-used. If you have some vitamin E capsules, one or two emptied into each bottle of oil that you use will help to stabilize the contents. You can buy oils which are rich in omega

3 and 6 in health food shops and these oils should be refrigerated and used within the recommended date and are not meant to be heated. Stir a couple of teaspoons of these oils into soups, pour on cooked food or add to salad dressings every day.

Fish

Whilst the larger, predatory fish such as tuna, salmon, shark, swordfish, sea bass and halibut and some bottom-feeding shellfish such as prawns provide a good source of omega 3 oils there are now concerns about the amount of methyl mercury they contain. The bigger the fish, the higher up the food chain and the longer it has lived, so one suggestion is not to eat fish larger than your plate (with the exception of salmon) and to be aware that fish steaks are cut from the larger fish. The smaller fish such as sardines, herring, small mackerel and anchovies still provide a good source of omega 3 oils with relatively little mercury contamination. A very simple and tasty fish paté can be made by processing smoked salmon or smoked mackerel with just a little melted butter and lemon juice and this also freezes very well. Aim to include oily fish in your diet several times a week. Occasionally, when you are mercury toxic and you unwittingly consume a food which contains high levels of methyl mercury such as seafood, you may experience vomiting or diarrhoea. This is known as a secondary immune reaction and is your body's way of eliminating the food and its associated toxins as quickly as possible.

Figure 16: Omega 3 oils and their actions

OMEGA 3 CHAIN

Alpha linolenic acid (ALA)
Sources: Plant sources such as flaxseed (55%), rape (10%), soy (8%), pumpkin, hemp, walnut, dark green leafy vegetables and oily fish.
Actions: Aids cardiovascular function. Some concern that it might promote prostate cancer.

Eicosapentanoic acid (EPA)
Sources: Oily fish.
Actions: Possibly the single most vital nutrient to brain and nerve function. Relieves depression, anxiety, feelings of guilt and worthlessness, insomnia and anxiety-related psychiatric disorders. Promotes cerebral blood flow and improves inter-neural communication which aids memory, learning and concentration. May actually aid regeneration of the brain.

Docosahexanoic acid (DHA)
Sources: Oily fish.
Actions: Probably most important during brain development and growth – a main component of the brain, nerves and eyes.

> # Figure 17: Food sources of minerals
>
> ### Magnesium
> Chocolate; nuts (almond, walnut, hazelnut, cashew, pistachio); green leafy vegetables; whole grains; seeds; pulses (beans, lentils); fruits (lemon, apple, orange, avocado, banana and fig); magnesium-rich salt and some mineral waters such as Badoit.
>
> ### Selenium
> Egg yolk; liver; kidney; cheddar cheese; butter; milk; scallops; smoked herring; tuna; brazil nuts; cashew nuts; wheat germ and bran; barley; brown rice; corn; oats; wholewheat bread; brewer's yeast; garlic; onion; kale; cabbage; broccoli; tomato and molasses.
>
> ### Zinc
> Beef; lamb; beef liver; egg yolk; chicken; sardines; oysters; herring; sunflower seeds; pumpkin seeds; brazil nuts; whole wheat; oats; almonds; banana; ginger; lentils and green peas.
>
> ### Calcium
> Nuts; seeds; pulses; tinned sardines; green leaves; dried apricots; raw cruciferous vegetables (cauliflower, cabbage, etc); hijuki seaweed.

Minerals

Toxic metals compete with minerals for binding sites and so a good mineral base is required to both displace the toxic metals and to replace them when they are dislodged by other means. Detoxification also requires a plentiful supply of a variety of minerals and these are often lacking in our modern diets. Try to incorporate mineral-rich foods into your diet and, since nutrients are always best when they come packaged in the way nature intended, juicing vegetables is a good way to obtain a plentiful supply of minerals in their natural form. FRS sufferers are frequently deficient in magnesium, selenium and zinc and figure 17 lists foods which are naturally rich in these minerals along with sources of calcium for those who may be avoiding dairy.

Celtic Sea Salt

Celtic Sea Salt is a source of trace minerals and should become the salt you use at the table and in cooking. Individuals suffering with adrenal fatigue actually *require salt* and often feel worse for consuming potassium-rich fruits and fruit juices which deplete sodium levels. You also need a certain amount of salt to synthesize stomach acid.

Prebiotics

These are foods which promote a healthy gut flora and include Jerusalem artichokes, soybeans, chicory root and raw oats, wheat and barley (if tolerated). Prebiotics aid mineral absorption, support the immune system and help to regulate bowel function, although their introduction may initially cause some intestinal upset. You can also use powdered Fructooligosaccharide (FOS), which is a prebiotic, as a sugar substitute.

The 'Bad' Foods

'Bad' Fats

'Bad' fats include the saturated fats found in meat, cheese, cream and lard. These fats promote inflammation and a surfeit also creates a relative deficiency of omega 3 oils which compete for the same enzymes. Try and reduce the frequency with which you eat meat and dairy products and/or reduce portion sizes. However, it is better to use small amounts of butter than any margarine (even if you are dairy-intolerant you may be able to tolerate butter).

Grapefruit

Grapefruit contains substances that are known to inhibit liver detoxification, so consider excluding or reducing intake of this fruit and its juice whilst you are ill.

Processed and Organ Meats

Consumption of processed meats such as bacon, sausages, corned beef, hot dogs and hamburgers should be kept to a minimum and any barbecued or burnt meat avoided wherever possible. Like us, animals store toxins in their body fat and their organs of excretion such as their liver and kidneys also become toxic so avoid organ meats and remove excess fat from meat where possible.

Sulphur-Containing Foods

Whilst sulphur is required for detoxification and inclusion of sulphur-rich foods and supplements is often recommended for FRS, experience shows that many sufferers find that consumption of these foodstuffs can prove problematic. This may be because sulphur is known to cause redistribution of mercury and to promote yeast growth in metal-toxic individuals, or may be due to the body vigorously detoxifying when supplied with sulphur-rich foods. If you find that one or more of these foods disagrees with you, you may wish to experiment with excluding *all* sulphur-containing foods and supplements for a while and reviewing your symptoms. Sulphur-rich foods include the cruciferous vegetables (broccoli, Brussels sprouts, cabbage, cauliflower, kale, kohlrabi, mustard, turnip and swede) in addition to peas, beans and their products, leeks, carob, chocolate, coffee, dairy products, eggs, lentils, Jerusalem artichokes, asparagus, onions, garlic, soy and its products, peanuts and spinach. Sulphur-containing supplements include: alpha-lipoic acid (ALA); chondroitin and glucosamine sulphate; glutathione; garlic; methylsulphonylmethane (MSM) and N-acetylcysteine (NAC).

The 'Ugly' Foods
Sugar Substitutes

Aspartame is the artificial sweetener used in a lot of diet products and soft drinks and marketed as NutraSweet, Equal, Spoonful or Equal Measure. As Russell Blaylock writes in his book *Excitoxins*, it acts as a neurotransmitter or 'excitotoxin' in the brain and in excess can literally stimulate nerve cells to death. Aspartame alone is responsible for *three-quarters* of all the complaints made to the powerful US Food and Drug Administration. It contains 50 per cent phenylalanine, 40 per cent aspartic acid and 10 per cent methanol. The phenylalanine is known to deplete serotonin levels in the brain causing depression and at body temperature the methanol breaks down into formic acid and formaldehyde which is highly toxic. Aspartame is recognized to cause nearly *one hundred symptoms* that can affect almost any body system and these include many of those that are familiar to FRS sufferers. However, the most consistent finding associated with Aspartame is that of memory loss.

High fructose corn syrup (HFCS) has been introduced in recent years to manufactured foods and drinks because it is both cheaper and twenty times sweeter than sugar. It now accounts for the majority of sweetener used, however it does not activate the insulin response, it encourages fat deposition and raises blood fats whilst failing to satiate and is thought to be a major cause of obesity. To add insult to injury, the majority of supplies are also mercury contaminated! There is also growing concern about the sweetener sucralose which is marketed as Splenda too – so scrutinize labels and eliminate all products containing artificial sweeteners.

Monosodium Glutamate

Monosodium glutamate (MSG) is also an excitotoxin which is added to a lot of savoury foods as a flavour enhancer. It can also be labelled as 'flavouring agents' or 'hydrolyzed vegetable protein' and is added to practically all ready meals, convenience foods, soups, snacks and nearly all fast foods. MSG causes such catastrophic metabolic and endocrine problems that it is used to induce obesity in experimental rats and mice. Cut out all products which contain – or might contain – MSG.

Hydrogenated and Trans-Fats

Hydrogenated fats will contain a proportion of trans-fats and both have been created by boiling vegetable oils under hydrogen in the presence of nickel to create hard fats that are cheap substitutes for butter. The trans-fats produced in this way have a different-shaped molecule and are completely synthetic, but the body mistakes them for naturally occurring oils and incorporates them into cell membranes where they impair various aspects of cell function. Eliminate hydrogenated oils or trans-fats completely, especially if you have fibromyalgia or a rapid respiration rate at rest. Look closely at labels because they are often an ingredient in manufactured foods such as biscuits (cookies), ice cream, cakes and sweets (candies). Note that both trans-fats and aspirin also block conversion of the good fats.

Special Diets

In addition to following the basic FRS diet, the specific dietary considerations required to manage food intolerances, overgrowth of Candida, hypoglycaemia, hypothyroidism and being overweight are addressed in more detail below. If your digestion is terribly compromised you also might want to consider using meal replacement powders such as Metagenic's Ultrameal to replace one or more meals a day. These do not need much digesting since they are a drink, supply a good balance of nutrients and largely eliminate the possibility of food intolerances.

Food Intolerances

The term intolerance is usually used to refer to foods that your body has difficulty digesting because you lack a particular enzyme, or refers to foods that have a detrimental effect upon your mental or physical processes in some way. This is in contrast to true food allergies which are usually more serious and more immediate. The symptoms caused by food intolerance tend to be delayed and more subtle and include migraines and headaches, behavioural and psychological changes, irritable bowel syndrome, asthma, eczema, rhinitis, rashes and catarrh. These symptoms also usually change throughout life so that many believe that they 'grew out of' a condition only to have the intolerance change its expression. Food intolerances can, however, change over time, so do not assume that because you once tested intolerant to a particular food you can never eat it again.

Identifying Food Intolerances

Your favourite foods often turn out to be the foods to which you are intolerant. This is because these foods have been creating a stress response which has been giving you a hormonal 'high' – whether you have been aware of it or not. You will certainly have been consciously or unconsciously including these foods in your diet every day or few days and may get cravings and withdrawal symptoms if you stop eating or drinking that particular foodstuff. The vast majority of FRS sufferers may have been controlled by these addictions and this may have played a large role in their developing chronic

---

Figure 18: Food intolerance testing methods

Blood test

York test or enzyme-linked immunosorbent assays (ELISA). A small sample of blood is taken and tested for reactions to proteins in food. This is relatively expensive, but may prove useful. Home test kits are now available.

Vega test

This is a machine that assesses the response of the energy meridians of the body to various foodstuffs and those having a detrimental effect are listed.

Muscle testing

Kinesiologists, allergy therapists and some nutritionists may use muscle testing to assess the response to vials containing foodstuffs. This is a more dynamic test than blood testing, as it can be reassessed on a regular basis.

---

fatigue. You may need to seek professional help in identifying food intolerances and figure 18 shows three of the more common methods of diagnosis.

DIY Food Intolerances

Without undertaking these tests, there is still much you can do to help yourself. The first suspects are the foods or drinks that you couldn't bear to give up – and they should be the first thing to go. Any foodstuff that you can't stop eating or drinking once you have started is also a sure-fire indication of intolerance and/or addiction. Please refer to figure 19 for a list of food groups which may help you identify foods from the same family that you may also need to avoid and to identify substitute foods in alternative food groups. There is often a family history of a particular food intolerance – so if you know that your uncle or grandmother was intolerant to dairy products, for instance, eliminating those would be a good place to start. Racial heredity also plays an important role, with the vast majority of adults of Asian descent being lactose intolerant. However, gluten intolerance is rare in people of Asian or African descent, but common in those with Celtic ancestry. Please note that some people who have problems with dairy may also need to exclude beef as they contain similar proteins.

Elimination Diets

Another DIY option is to go on a restricted diet for a short period of time with the intention of eliminating the most likely allergens and then reintroducing them one by one and gauging the reaction. Options include:

- Eating the healthy Stone Age diet outlined previously, but cutting out all dairy products and gluten-containing grains because these two foodstuffs are responsible for the lion's share of intolerances. The grains that contain gluten

Figure 19: Food groups

Fruit families	Foods
Apple	Apple, pear, quince
Banana	Arrowroot, banana, plantain
Beech	Beechnut, chestnut
Birch	Cobnuts, hazelnuts, filberts
Blueberry	Blueberry, cranberry
Cashew	Cashew nut, mango, pistachio
Citrus	Clementine, grapefruit, lemon, lime, mandarin, orange, satsuma, tangerine, ugly
Gourd	Cantaloupe, courgette (zucchini), cucumber, gherkin, honeydew melon, pumpkin, squash, watermelon
Grape	Brandy, champagne, cream of tartar, currants, sherry, sultanas, raisins, wine
Plum	Almond, apricot, cherry, peach, plum
Palm	Coconut, date, sago
Rose	Blackberry, loganberry, raspberry, rosehip, sloe, strawberry
NO relatives	Black pepper, Brazil nut, fig, juniper, kiwi fruit, lychee, maple, olive, papaya, pawpaw, pecan, pineapple, sesame, tea, vanilla, walnut

Vegetable families	Foods
Buckwheat	Buckwheat, rhubarb
Composite	Artichoke, burdock, camomile, chicory, dandelion, lettuce, safflower, sunflower
Fungi and moulds	Baker's yeast, brewer's yeast, mushrooms, truffles, cheese, vinegar
Goosefoot (beet)	Beet, chard, spinach, sugar beet
Grasses	Bamboo shoots, barley, cane sugar, corn, millet, oats, rice, rye, wheat
Laurel	Avocado, cinnamon
Lily	Asparagus, chives, garlic, leeks, onions, shallot
Mint	Mint, basil, marjoram, oregano, sage, rosemary, thyme
Mustard	Broccoli, Brussels sprouts, cabbage, cauliflower, cress, horseradish, kohlrabi, mustard, radish, swede, turnip, watercress
Nightshade	Aubergine (eggplant), cape gooseberry, chilli, paprika, peppers, potato, tobacco, tomato
Parsley	Anise, caraway, carrot, celery, coriander, cumin, dill, fennel, parsley, parsnip
Pulses and legumes	Alfalfa, chickpea, haricot beans, kidney beans, lentils, liquorice, mung beans, pea, peanut, soya bean (TVP), string beans, tamarind
Sterculia	Chocolate, cocoa, cola nut
NO relatives	Ginseng, coffee, sweet potato, yam

Animal families	Foods
Bovine	Beef, dairy, goat, lamb, milk, mutton
Poultry	Chicken, egg, pheasant, quail
Duck	Duck, goose
Swine	Bacon, pork, ham, lard, sausage
Flatfish	Dab, flounder, halibut, plaice, sole, turbot
Salmon	Salmon, trout
Mackerel	Mackerel, tuna
Codfish	Cod, coley, haddock, hake
Herring	Herring, pilchard, rollmop, sardine
Molluscs	Abalone, clam, mussel, oyster, scallop, snail, squid
Crustacean	Crab, crayfish, lobster, prawns, shrimp
NO relatives	Anchovy, caviar, rabbit, turkey, venison

include wheat, rye, oats and barley and these can be replaced with gluten-free grains such as millet, quinoa (pronounced keen-wa), buckwheat, rice and corn/maize (although corn is a common allergen too). When excluding dairy products cut out all milk, yoghurt, cream, crème fraiche, butter and cheese and check that products do not include dairy products in any form.

- Another alternative is to cut out the 'sensitive seven' most likely allergens which are: dairy products, wheat, sugar, corn, soy and its products, eggs and peanuts. The second tier allergens include: yeast, oranges, tomatoes, coffee, citrus fruits, beef, pork, potato, nuts, tea and chocolate. You could cut both tiers out and then re-introduce the second tier allergens first one by one, observing any symptoms.
- You can just eat lamb, pears and rice (you are very unlikely to be intolerant to these foods) for a few days. Alternatively, you can try eating a diet of exotic foods that you rarely eat such as rabbit, duck, lobster, kiwi fruit, pineapple, mango, and so on for a limited time as these foods are unlikely to be the culprits – or do a bit of both!
- Testing foods using the techniques described in the appendix may also be helpful.
- Another alternative is to try a powdered meal replacement such as Metagenics' Ultrameal (dairy free) for a few days, although you should probably supplement this with some plain meat or fish.

It is quite normal when you eliminate a food to which you are intolerant to experience some quite severe withdrawal symptoms. These may include migraines, headaches and flu-like symptoms and typically occur within a few days, but may take weeks to manifest. You may also find that when you reintroduce the food, you may get an extreme reaction that you did not get when your body was habitually exposed to it. Some people also find that they lose a lot of water weight when they eliminate a food to which they are intolerant and may find that they bloat up when they consume the food again.

Reintroducing Foods

- Introduce foods one by one, keeping a food diary. Sometimes symptoms are not immediate so include aches, sleep patterns and headaches over the following few days.
- Choose the simplest, plainest form of any food. For instance, if reintroducing oats, try making oatmeal porridge with water and not eating an oat biscuit or cookie where any reaction could be to the other ingredients.

- You could monitor your heart rate and blood pressure an hour or two after eating to gauge a reaction, with any great increases in either measurement indicating a food intolerance.
- To confuse the situation even more, some sufferers are able to tolerate modest amounts of some foods on an occasional basis. However, if they have a food they tolerated on day one again on day two, they may have a reaction. For this reason, some people deliberately rotate ingredients in a four- or five-day cycle in order to avoid a reaction. Some food intolerances also seem to come and go and this may relate to how much mercury is in circulation at any given time. If you have periodically been able to tolerate a foodstuff during recovery, the ability to eat that food *will* return permanently if you keep going with the detoxification.

The Anti-Candida Diet

If you suspect that you have an overgrowth of Candida albicans (see figure 2) then you may need to stick to a strict anti-Candida diet until your symptoms have improved. Be warned, though, Candida converts into its cyst form when food supplies are scarce and can remain in this dormant state for years until foods are reintroduced. The anti-Candida diet is essentially the Stone Age diet but with particular emphasis on avoiding alcohol, refined carbohydrates, sugar, dairy, yeast and fungi. Please see figure 20 for a list of the foods that need to be eliminated according to the severity of your condition. Desserts are out – but you can have fruit after a few weeks and you may find that you tolerate berries better than other fruits. Treating candidal overgrowth by diet alone is treating a symptom rather than the cause – although it may provide essential management for a period of time. When you feel that you may have re-established control, you can start to reintroduce some foods one at a time, cautiously observing symptoms. When Candida dies it can produce an unpleasant Herxheimer (die-off) reaction and/or crashing cravings for its preferred foodstuffs and these are actually encouraging signs that what you are doing is working and furthermore that Candida is an underlying problem. Once you have weathered these storms, you may start to feel quite a lot better than you have felt in a long time. There are many books devoted exclusively to this subject and any natural health practitioner will be able to help you.

Figure 20: Foods to avoid for control of candidal overgrowth

Category	Foods
Moderate	
Fermented foods	All alcohol (especially wine and beer); vinegar; citric acid; pickles; soy sauce and tofu.
Yeast-based products	Marmite; yeast extract (often added – look at the label); blue cheese; yeast-containing stock cubes or powder; brewer's yeast; yeast-containing supplements – especially B vitamins and selenium; anything malted; mushrooms; truffles.
Sugar	Treacle; syrup; molasses; honey; fructose; maltose; glucose; sorbitol; molasses; date sugar or maple sugar. All artificial sweeteners should also be avoided although Xylitol and Agave syrup are natural sweeteners that can be used in moderation.
Serious	
Refined carbohydrates	Anything made with flour including: pies; pasta; crackers; pastries; cakes; crumpets; biscuits; cookies; doughnuts and muffins. Bread is both a refined carbohydrate and yeast-containing and should be avoided completely.
Dairy products	Milk; buttermilk; butter; cream; sour cream; crème fraiche, cottage cheese and cheese are all favoured foodstuffs of Candida.
Severe	
Fruit	If very severe, avoid fruit completely, otherwise eat no more than one or two portions of fresh fruit a day, peel the fruit and avoid melon and fruit that has a bloom (yeast) such as plums or grapes. Do not eat dried fruit either for a while, as this is very high in sugar and yeast.
Nuts	Only eat nuts that you have cracked yourself, otherwise you can probably eat modest quantities of nuts (make sure that they are as fresh as possible because they can get mouldy).

Figure 21: Goitrogenic and beneficial foods for hypothyroidism

Category	Foods
Goitrogenic foods	
Cruciferous vegetables	Broccoli; Brussels sprouts; cabbage; cauliflower; kale; kohlrabi; mustard; rutabaga; turnip and swede.
Soybean and products	Tofu; tempeh; soy sauce; soy milk and textured vegetable protein (TVP).
Miscellaneous food	Strawberries; peaches; millet; corn (maize); peanuts; almonds; walnuts; pine nuts; cassava; radishes and spinach.
Beneficial foods	
Tyrosine-containing foods	Avocado; pumpkin and sesame seeds; cashew nuts; banana and dairy.
Iodine-containing foods	Algae (kelp); iodized salt; shellfish; sea fish; sardines; radish; onion; mushroom; turnip; pineapple; egg white and cheddar cheese.

The Hypoglycaemia Diet

Eating a diet that regulates your blood sugar levels is a very important part of recovery. This means eating according to the glycaemic index or glycaemic load of foods (GI/GL index), which is a measure of the impact that specific foods have on your blood sugar levels. There are many books devoted exclusively to this subject.

In brief, the rules for low GI eating are:

- Cut out all sweet and refined foods.
- Cut down or cut out consumption of alcohol and fruit juices.
- Substitute xylitol (a naturally low GI sweetener) for sugar.
- Eat smaller meals regularly and do not skip meals – especially breakfast.
- Eat whole foods as much as possible.
- Root vegetables (excluding potatoes) are a good source of slow releasing carbohydrates.
- Eat low GI fruits such as apples, apricots, berries, cherries, citrus fruits, pears and plums.
- Try to combine proteins and carbohydrates in both snacks (hummus on oatcakes) and meals (fish or meat and vegetables).
- Finally, consuming a protein drink with meals may help to regulate your blood sugar.

The Hypothyroidism Diet

If you have an underactive thyroid gland, then it might be best to avoid consuming foods known as goitrogens which interfere with the synthesis of thyroxine and can cause a swelling of the gland known as a goitre. The jury is still out as to how much harm some of these foods do in practice, and cooking may deactivate some of the components, however it would be wise to avoid inclusion of excessive amounts of the goitrogenic foods in the diet. Equally, the body requires both the amino acid tyrosine and the trace element iodine to synthesize thyroxine, and so foods containing these compounds are beneficial to thyroid function and should be included (within reason) in the diet. Foods in both categories are listed in figure 21.

The Weight-Loss Diet

Other books will confidently inform you that regular exercise combined with a healthy diet will result in weight loss. My experience is that (depending upon your particular toxicity or endocrine dysfunction) excess weight cannot only prove damnably hard to shift, but impossible for some with FRS. Certainly don't be tempted into using extreme or damaging measures such as fad diets, diuretics, abusing laxatives or surgery.

Consider the following possibilities if stubborn excess weight is an issue for you.

- If you have an untreated or inadequately treated underactive thyroid gland, it will be impossible to lose weight. Some of those with hypothyroidism may have metabolisms which are running at 50 or 70 per cent of the ideal. The thyroid gland also starts to produce reverse T3 (rT3) when food is restricted and this mechanism can reduce the metabolic rate by a further 30 per cent, meaning that you literally can't eat little enough to lose weight without starvation. It is probably a survival strategy and may also be the mechanism by which dieting makes you fat. You are effectively warning your body that food may occasionally be scarce and to conserve supplies. Certainly consult a doctor and/or naturopath if weight loss is all but impossible or you are getting bigger in spite of all your best efforts to lose weight.
- Ensure that you have identified *all* your food intolerances and that you strictly avoid these foods.
- Toxin levels in fat can be up to 1,000 times higher than those in the blood and if you are still very toxic your body will refuse to release fat from storage and even if it does, the fat typically becomes dimpled and reforms the minute you resume eating anything approaching a normal diet. This is why cellulite is so hard to get rid of and why you may feel a whole lot worse if you do manage to lose weight as you experience a toxin surge. Do the best that you can and keep detoxifying.
- Kidney damage may also mean that you are retaining a lot of water and this will eventually be resolved by detoxification.
- Some people, particularly those who may have had childhood experiences of sexual abuse, may be running a subconscious programme that being overweight provides some sort of protection. If this is the case, no amount of work on the physical will override this programme for very long. If you think that this might be true for you, then seek the help of a specialist practitioner who can access the subconscious and re-programme this belief. Therapies such as PSYCH-K, kinesiology or Emotional Freedom Technique can be particularly valuable in this regard.
- Historic loss of a child can profoundly impact blood sugar management and be the underlying cause of morbid obesity or enormous struggles with weight and this applies to men as well as women. Again, you may need to seek help to resolve this underlying issue in order to lose weight.

Fasting

Fasting may seem like an appealing way of rapidly detoxifying and losing weight, but fasting is best reserved for maintenance of health in essentially well people for several reasons. First, starvation is a huge stress to the body and taxes potentially exhausted adrenal and thyroid glands yet further. Second, as fat stores are broken down, the toxins stored are released at the same time as the body is deprived of the nutrients and energy it requires to detoxify them. Third, fasting also induces greater phase I detoxification in the liver which means that highly toxic substances are generated that cannot then be further processed because the cofactors required for phase II detoxification are absent. Fourth, with a complete lack of fibre, toxins excreted in the bile will be reabsorbed. Last but not least, the complete lack of dietary antioxidants means that there will be more reactive oxygen species damage occurring throughout the body.

Fluids

> The cell is immortal. It is merely the fluid in which if floats that degenerates. Renew this fluid at regular intervals, give the cells what they require for nutrition, and as far as we know, the pulsation of life can go on forever.
>
> **Dr Alexis Carell**

We are about 75 per cent water by weight and 99 per cent of the molecules in our bodies are water molecules. Next to oxygen, water is the most vital substance for sustaining life and dehydration is the most threatening stress to any living thing. Adequate water supplies are essential for efficient blood and lymph flow, the production of digestive juices, the prevention of constipation, kidney function, cushioning and lubricating the joints and intervertebral discs and for the efficient function of the brain. Most people in the developed world are chronically dehydrated because most of the preferred beverages cause a net loss of water over time. Many only drink when they feel thirsty too, when thirst is really an alarm signalling dehydration. Even just existing, we need to replace the 2 litres (3.5 pints) of water a day that are lost through sweating, moisture in our breath, urinating, tears, defecating and menstruating. Chronic dehydration can manifest as the symptoms of many different illnesses that often then get treated with medication. Whilst we come equipped with an efficient drought management system that ensures that the vital organs always have the constant supply of water they require in order for us to survive, constant flushing of the intercellular fluid and kidneys is vital to recovery in the mercury-toxic individual.

What to Drink

Try to avoid drinks that contain sugar, caffeine, any kind of colouring or preservative, or dairy (if you are dairy intolerant). Caffeinated drinks are not only dehydrating, but also stress your overworked adrenal glands and kidneys. Many people with FRS may not tolerate fruit juices or smoothies very well because they deplete sodium reserves, present a big challenge to your blood sugar control mechanism and promote the overgrowth of Candida. In addition to the declared chemical constituents, canned drinks are often made using fluoridated water and may contain traces of both Bisphenol A and the metal used in the can. Basically, whilst you can enjoy a variety of herbal teas and some fruit and vegetable juices, the majority of the time you need to be drinking *room-temperature water*.

Whilst tap water is usually hygienic, it may contain chlorine, fluorine, herbicides, pesticides, pharmaceuticals and various toxic metals. Ideally, your domestic supply of water for drinking and cooking should either be bottled or processed using a reverse osmosis filter and once installed, these provide a plentiful supply of pure water relatively cheaply. Simple carbon jug filters are cheap and better than nothing and even leaving water to stand in a wide-necked glass jug (preferably on a windowsill in the sun) allows much of the chlorine to evaporate. Adding a couple of grains of Celtic Sea Salt to each litre of water drunk can also help to provide the trace minerals that your body requires without making the water salty. Some mineral waters (such as Badoit) are particularly high in magnesium and other minerals and may be of benefit, however, plasticizers from plastic bottles can contaminate the water, so buy your water in glass bottles where possible. Be careful to check the labels of any healthy-looking flavoured waters, which often contain chemical flavourings and sweeteners. It is a good idea to devise a system for making sure you are consistently drinking adequate amounts of water by, for example, filling a bottle in the morning and drinking it throughout the day. Whilst drinking too much water too quickly is counterproductive, even when you are drinking plentiful supplies it may take months for the effects of chronic dehydration to reverse. Try also to avoid drinking with meals as this dilutes your digestive juices – although drinking mineral water with a meal has been shown to increase magnesium uptake.

There are also specific water products that aim to promote hydration and electrolyte balance, and water that has been alkalinized and energized in various ways, and these may also help. Finally, Masaru Emoto developed a technique of photographing the ice crystals formed by water from different sources treated in different ways and these are illustrated in his books such as *The Hidden Messages in Water*. Some of the most beautiful crystals produced relate to water that has been blessed and may shed some light on the old wisdom of blessing your food and drink before consuming it.

Alcohol Intolerance

A lot of people with FRS become alcohol intolerant, especially to the alcohol produced from grapes and grains which includes such drinks as wine, bitter, lager, whisky, brandy and sherry. This is most probably because overgrowth of Candida has depleted the liver of all the nutrients required to process alcohol. As a result, even having just a tiny amount of wine can make some FRS sufferers feel hung-over and generally unwell the next day – or for several days afterwards. You may find that you can tolerate modest amounts of spirits such as tequila (made from cactus); gin (juniper berries); rum (sugar cane); sake (rice); Campari (secret formula – but seems OK) and any spirit made from other fruits such as Cointreau (oranges), Limoncello (lemons) or Dubonnet (blackcurrants). Some can also tolerate champagne because it is double-fermented and lower in yeast than wine. Basically though, your liver is struggling to detoxify alcohol and the signs that this is particularly true for you include getting hot, sweaty or restless between 1 and 3am or being wakeful during these hours. If you have insomnia then alcohol, along with other stimulating drinks such as coffee or cola, should be the first thing to go. Alcohol only gives the impression of helping you to go to sleep, but actually profoundly disrupts your sleep patterns and may leave you restless after a few hours of unconsciousness.

Chapter 15

Emotional Work

Turn your wounds into wisdom.

Oprah Winfrey

You can follow the FRS diet and take every supplement recommended and still fail to improve if you hate your father for leaving when you were a child or loathe your job. You absolutely have to sort out as much emotional baggage as you possibly can, especially the burning issues – and for the most part, you will know what they are. Any anger, grievances, resentments, regrets and guilt will keep you sick, or at least keep you from being fully well. You need to work through it all and do it completely because your life literally depends upon it.

Work

Surveys show that up to 85 per cent of people don't like their jobs and yet we spend such a huge amount of our lives at work that it is important to your health and well-being that you like what you do for a living. You may know that you have to work to pay the mortgage and utility bills, but in getting an FRS, your soul and your body may have found their own way of objecting to a job you dislike. Sometimes the solution is closer at hand than you imagine, for instance, offering to job share or be transferred to another department, requesting flexi-time, reducing or changing your work hours or working from home one day a week may make things more tolerable. It might also be possible to take early retirement, a leave of absence or a sabbatical of some sort. If you really hate your job or the people at your place of work, then handing in your notice might be the right thing for you to do, however, don't take any precipitous decisions without thinking them through first. What if you are ill for a lot longer than you currently imagine is likely? How are you going to afford to get better, because it does take money? Certainly investigate what rights you may have accrued in your current job and then make a considered and informed decision about the best way forward.

> **Diseases can be our spiritual flat tyres – disruptions in our lives that seem to be disasters at the time but end by redirecting our lives in a meaningful way.**
>
> **Dr Bernie Siegel**

It may be that your soul and the universe are forcing you off your current trajectory in order to ultimately get you onto a more fulfilling career track. Is there something else you have always wanted to do? If you knew that you had six months to live or if you won the lottery, what would you do? Is it possible for you to do that now or to take one step on the path towards doing it? Even knowing that there is a light at the end of the tunnel can make a considerable difference to the way you feel in the present.

Look On the Bright Side

> **If only people knew the healing power of laughter and joy, many of our fine doctors would be out of business.**
>
> **Catherine Ponder**

Life can get very serious when you are chronically sick. The world truly is a madhouse and footage of the most horrific and tragic events occurring in the world are broadcast directly into your living room several times a day. Consider having a news blackout for a while, or certainly only watch the news headlines once a day and preferably not immediately before going to bed. Now may also not be the best time to watch gritty documentaries about the holocaust or blockbuster films about disasters.

On the other hand, laughter is great medicine so make a point of reading amusing books, listening to comedy, watching funny films or TV programmes and going to see a favourite comedian. If you haven't done so before, start to value and treat yourself in whatever way is meaningful to you. Go out for a meal, have a bath or massage or read a novel. It is also worth incorporating some form of contemplation or quiet time into your life and this may mean a walk in the woods, listening to beautiful music, meditating or some kind of worship. Feed your soul by doing things that you used to enjoy or have always wanted to do, but may have put on the back burner for later in your life. Any changes that you make in your life – even minor ones – change the dynamic and will start to produce different results.

Learning to Say 'No'

Almost everyone wants to be liked and this is a particular issue for women who want to be thought of as 'nice' and so often end up agreeing to things when they really should have refused. The trouble is that whilst everyone else may or may not think well of you, you end up despising yourself, not living the life you would choose and your body ends up saying 'No' for you. You can't be all things to all people. They will get by just fine without you and they might have to, if you don't get well!

Energy Drains

Sometimes we have historically formed dependent emotional ties to others or they to us and these connections can unwittingly and unknowingly be draining our energies. These bonds are usually with people that we love or have loved – a parent or an ex-partner or even someone who has subsequently died. In these cases, it may be necessary for you to do some inner work on symbolically releasing and severing those ties. We can also have formed other draining and more esoteric energetic attachments, often when we were vulnerable, and it can take someone conversant in dealing with these matters to resolve them.

Other People

Many people with FRS become introverted and find being with other people a particular drain. Think carefully about who lifts you up and makes you feel positive and strong and, conversely, who drains you and leaves you feeling less good about yourself – even if you ostensibly like them. Try to reduce or eliminate contact with the latter and nourish the supportive friendships. FRS is a great test of relationships and you may find that you emerge from this experience with a completely different set of friends and a different attitude. You probably don't still have the same group of friends you had when you were a child or teenager, so allow non-supportive friendships to fade into the background. Mercury toxicity specifically affects interpersonal skills, whereby you may have difficulty interpreting others' meaning and motivations and you may also unwittingly upset them. When I was really fighting for my life, friends got upset with me about things that I considered to be fantastically trivial. The thing to remember at these times is that in other people's eyes you probably don't look anywhere near as sick as you feel and it is hard for them to appreciate just how ill you may be.

Figuring It Out

It may be worth asking some gentle questions of family or friends and trying to piece together events in your childhood or family history in general. Try to do this in as casual a manner as possible and make sure that your questions imply no accusation or blame – you are simply trying to understand some of what may have occurred from an adult perspective. People may become defensive anyway if there is something to hide and you may meet a wall of denial, because groups have a way of trying to protect themselves whilst also trying to manage a young child's memories. They may have concluded that by not talking about an event or indeed, by even denying it ever occurred, the child is spared some of the trauma. It may have been well-intentioned, but effectively the child's future mental and physical health may have been sacrificed by this strategy.

You may ultimately feel that you cannot heal without confronting others and this has to be your decision. A word of warning though: sometimes individuals feel more traumatized by the denials and recriminations that follow than by the original event. It may not be possible to confront or even question any of the parties involved, because you may no longer be in contact with them, or they may be dead or senile, in which case you will have to resolve the matter as best you can. Ultimately, this is for you and it is about changing *your* attitude to what has happened – you don't need to recruit anyone else to do that.

To have become a deeper man is the privilege of those who have suffered.

Oscar Wilde

Families

Many FRS sufferers' illnesses may have been initiated earlier in their life by dysfunctional family relationships and these can continue to be a chronic source of stress. Try to address these in the best way you can, which may mean having to tackle touchy subjects such as telling your parents that you are planning a quiet Christmas at home this year. Don't ask that they be happy about the changes that you may need to make, just that they accept them. For those with severe FRS, your life may literally be on the line (which is not going to be something that others will acknowledge or understand) and this knowledge can make you square up to issues that you may have previously been reluctant to address. Some family relationships really can't be fixed and sometimes it is just better to recognize that fact and then work hard to prevent the same toxic patterns being handed down to the next generation. Severing all ties with family members may be appropriate in some circumstances, however I would recommend less drastic action wherever possible.

Useful Therapies

If you gave some thought to the emotional issues raised in chapter 11, you may have been able to piece together the events that you think may have played a role in your FRS. The more you can sort through and release these often historic feelings, the more you will be able to release toxic deposits of all kinds held within your body. You will most probably require some form of outside help in order to do this. Talking therapies are useful and you may resolve quite a lot of issues in this way, however, they do not address what is beyond conscious recall for which you may need to try hypnotherapy. There are also different kinds of bodywork that may help to release issues held in the body such as deep tissue massage and Rolfing. A book entitled *The Journey* by Brandon Bays has given rise to intensive courses of the same name which can also release early traumas. Rebirthing breathwork sessions with a therapist may also be effective and are not exclusively related to recalling birth trauma as the name might imply. It is also very supportive of your physical detoxification to supplement using vibrational remedies such as Bach flower remedies throughout treatment (see chapter 17). If you can find a kinesiologist in your area who addresses the emotional aspects of illness, they may also be able to unearth issues that may be affecting you. 'Constellation therapy', as developed by Bert Hellinger, also helps to address wider family issues and the possibility of having taken on suffering that is not yours – if you suspect that this might be the case. In any event, there are all sorts of courses and therapists available if you look for them who may be able to help you on your healing journey.

Doing It Yourself

If you do not want to, or cannot afford to get professional help, there is still a lot you can do for yourself. The only issue is that you might let yourself off the hook in a way that a therapist might not. Get curious. Ask yourself all sorts of questions such as: Were you planned? Was your arrival greeted with joy, fear, disappointment or shame? Are you sure that you are actually the child of the parents you imagine are yours? Had your parents wanted a child of the opposite gender? What was going on in your family at the time of your birth? Were your parents getting on? Was your father away a lot? It is quite common for one or both parents to have had affairs at some point, which they probably tried to hide, but children are acutely perceptive. They may not understand the adult world, but they do sense everything. Could this have happened when you were younger? Try reconstructing the time line of your life by writing about various dated events and filling in the blanks as memories resurface. It is surprising what you may start to remember when you begin this process. For more help on this subject, John Bradshaw's book *Family Secrets: What you don't know can hurt you* is an instructive guide to sorting through family dysfunction, and *Love's Hidden Symmetry* by Bert Hellinger addresses roles within the family over the previous two generations.

You could find and frame pictures of the young you and send this little person your love or write to them offering support and encouragement. You might also want to try writing letters to various people and then creating a ceremony to burn them. This only works if you let it all out, really express what you feel and don't hold back. You could also try building a visualization around imagining the 'cords' that may have kept you tied to others being severed. If you can find it in your heart, thank them for the part they have played in your journey and release these ties with love. Various forms of energy tapping are also very effective at releasing old emotions and there are many books available on this subject. You may want to go into the middle of nowhere and have a good scream or beat pillows, cry, bang drums – anything that lets emotions out. You may want to put up a punch bag in the spare room or garage and release pent-up emotions that way. Alternatively, you may find it therapeutic to draw or paint issues or feelings or do some kind of storyboard using pictures from magazines. Try also 'catching' the endless babble of your inner dialogue and asking, 'Now where has that come from?' You could also try journaling – that is keeping an occasional 'emotional' diary and possibly trying to recall and write down any dreams too.

It is no measure of health to be well adjusted to a profoundly sick society.

Krishnamurti

The Big Picture

For my money all this forgiving is hard to do completely until you understand that we all come round again and again on the wheel of life and we all play different parts. This is what half the population of this planet believes, although it is not part of the modern Judeo-Christian tradition that predominates in the developed world. We form soul contracts with various others to experience certain aspects of the human condition and as hard as this may be to believe, *this is done with the express agreement of our soul for our greater spiritual development*. So you see everyone was just playing the part in your life that your soul agreed they needed to play – be that bully, rapist, fraudster or unfaithful partner. Ultimately, there really aren't any victims and no one is to blame. You also need to accept that you are not perfect and that you have, possibly unknowingly, done others harm for which they may still feel aggrieved. Allied with this is the fact that some of the issues that we come into this life to address are carried over from other lifetimes. For this reason, sometimes it can be therapeutic to explore the past life background to a particular conflict or problematic relationship using hypnosis or regression. There are also books and CDs available for home use such as *Healing Your Past Lives* by Roger Woolger which may be helpful.

> **Forgiveness, love and our connection with the Divine is the medicine that is healing the sickness of our time.**
>
> **J Artos Roske**

Coping

Typically, most FRS sufferers have difficulties with their memory which will improve with detoxification – along with all other cognitive functions. In the meantime, make lists and notes by keeping a little pad handy at all times. Do things straight away as much as you can and then not only do you not have to remember the task, but also you are not haunted by the thought that there is something you have forgotten. Develop simple systems for paying bills such as writing a cheque on receipt and putting it in a dated envelope to be sent later or, alternatively, arrange to pay everything by direct debit where possible. Simplify your life as much as you can. In the words of the architect and designer William Morris, 'Have nothing in your house that you do not know to be useful, or believe to be beautiful.' If you haven't worn it, read it, listened to it or watched it in over a year – you don't need it. Sell it, give it to someone who will enjoy it or give it to charity. Then sort out and order what remains. Develop routines and put things in the same places and demand that others do. These actions symbolically clear the past and create the space for you to move forward into (hopefully) a bright new future.

Chapter 16

Lifestyle

> As I see it, every day you do one of two things: build
> health or produce disease in yourself.
>
> **Adelle Davis**

This chapter examines the various aspects of lifestyle that need to be embraced or eliminated in order to recover from FRS. First, we turn our attention to the important issue of sleep (or lack of it), which for a great many sufferers is probably the most persistent and troublesome aspect of the disorder.

Sleep

> Sleep is the golden chain that ties health and our bodies together.
>
> **Thomas Dekker**

Many FRS sufferers experience difficulty getting to sleep, are wakeful in the night, wake very early or awaken feeling tired and 'drugged'. Deep sleep is when the body repairs and renews, when antibodies are produced, when the liver does the majority of its work and when memories are stored and so good-quality sleep is absolutely vital for recovery from FRS. Being unable to sleep is incredibly frustrating and there is nothing lonelier that keeping a solitary vigil throughout the night, night after night, when everyone else appears to be sleeping. In fact, the sleep aid market doubled in the five years to 2007, so insomnia is unfortunately a growing modern-day problem and you are *definitely* not alone.

The pineal gland (the 'third eye') has light receptors similar to the eye and communicates with the hypothalamus, which regulates all the other endocrine organs, and it is thought to be responsible for initiating puberty and the menopause and ageing in general. The pineal gland converts serotonin into melatonin during the hours of darkness and greatly reduced amounts during the hours of daylight. Serotonin is produced in a two-step process from the essential amino acid tryptophan consumed in the diet to 5-hydroxytryptophan (5-HTP), which is then converted into serotonin. Quite apart from regulating sleep/wake cycles, melatonin is a potent general antioxidant that specifically acts within the central nervous system.

The following suggestions may help if lack of sleep is an issue for you:

- Make sure that your bedroom is a place of rest by having a good clear out, removing any televisions and computers and redecorating if necessary. Remove all electrical appliances from around the head of the bed as discussed in chapter 13. Your room needs to be dark at night to promote melatonin production so put up black-out blinds if necessary and eliminate any sources of light within the room. An alarm clock that slowly lights up before going off will help to convert melatonin into serotonin before you wake and may help if you struggle to wake up or feel dreadful in the mornings.
- Make sure that the temperature and ventilation in the room are comfortable and you may need different layers of bedding that can be added and removed as required. If you find that you have difficulty sleeping in your own bed but sleep better elsewhere, consider either changing the bed if it has a metal frame, buying a good quality mattress or moving the bed. If it is a snoring partner or other noises that disturb or wake you, first try foam earplugs. Alternatively, white noise machines can drown out some background noise or you may need to sleep in another room if this is possible.
- Establish a calming routine by having a bath with a few drops of lavender and/or chamomile essential oil added whilst listening to music and then making for bed early and reading a slightly heavy-going book. Short naps in the daytime might be restorative, but set an alarm for 40 minutes at the most and if you find it is interfering with your sleep at night, then cut it out. If sleep is absolutely impossible, then at least lie down and relax for some of the night because the body requires you to be horizontal in order to do much of its repair work.
- Try to do some form of exercise every day and to get outdoors – if only briefly – as both these activities help regulate sleep cycles. Light boxes and light visors are also available and are intended for use primarily in the dark days of winter to relieve seasonal affective disorder, but may also help to regulate sleep.
- Some pharmaceutical drugs can adversely affect sleep so consider trying alternatives or attempting to wean yourself off any tablets with your doctor's permission or knowledge if you think this might be the case. This can be hard and you may need to set aside a couple of weeks' holiday and just accept that

your sleep will be erratic for a little while whilst your body re-establishes its own rhythm.

- If pain or discomfort is the primary reason for sleeplessness, then a Tempur foam mattress or mattress cover may help to distribute pressure. Ultimately, the lesser of two evils might be to take painkillers to ensure a decent night's sleep. Magnets can also be used therapeutically and there are many magnetic products available including mattress covers, blankets, bracelets, straps and bandages. Alternatively, you can experiment with taping a flat disc-shaped magnet to body parts or sewing it into pyjamas. The north-seeking pole strengthens and stimulates and the south-seeking pole sedates, relaxes and can be used for pain relief. Muscle testing will help you to identify what works (see the Appendix).

- The food and drink you consume can be a major source of sleeplessness, so eliminate all stimulants, such as tobacco, tea, coffee, alcohol, colas, sugar, cheese, aspartame and monosodium glutamate (MSG). If you can feel your heart hammering at night or your blood pressure or heart rate are increased and this is associated with loose bowel movements or diarrhoea the next day, the chances are that you are reacting to something you have eaten. Supplementing digestive enzymes with all meals and avoiding eating any foods that you may be intolerant to may help. If you do occasionally react to foods in this way, two to four capsules of a supplement such as BioCare's Bio-carbonate capsules will normally quell the reaction within half an hour or so, enabling you to sleep. This can be useful after eating out on the occasions when you may not have been able to control which foods you have eaten, but should not be relied upon on as a means of management on an on-going basis. To assess whether food intolerances are playing a major part in your insomnia, you could try just consuming a meal replacement product such as Metagenics' Ultrameal for a few days and drinking water. If you sleep like a baby, then food intolerances may be playing a large part in your sleeplessness. Please refer to chapter 14 for more information on identifying food intolerances.

- If you find that you wake in the night to urinate and have difficulty getting back to sleep, try reducing fluids in the hours before bedtime. If you do need to go to the toilet, try to remember your dream, avoid putting any lights on (as this will shut down melatonin production instantly) and try to 'continue' the dream you were having to aid return to sleep.

- Some foods are particularly rich in tryptophan, from which melatonin is ultimately synthesized, and including them in your diet may help to regulate both mood and sleep. Tryptophan-rich foods include tofu and most soy products, black-eyed peas, walnuts and almonds, sesame and roasted pumpkin seeds and turkey. Chamomile tea drunk several times throughout the day and at bedtime can also help to induce sleep.

- Feeling restless, wakeful or hot between one and three o'clock in the morning is a strong indication that your liver is struggling. If this is a time when you are often sleepless, you may need to clean up your diet, cut out all alcohol and take a supplement to aid liver function. Sometimes too, your body just does not seem to be able to 'turn off'. This may be because you are not breaking down adrenaline and noradrenaline (epinephrine and norepinephrine) properly, and taking a little of a product such as Metagenics' Ultraclear Sustain before bed may enable sleep.
- Underlying candidal or parasitic infections are also a common cause of insomnia and you may need to enlist the help of a natural therapist to eliminate these issues.
- The presence of mercury in circulation appears to cause a profound insomnia and because you are deliberately mobilizing mercury out of storage in order to excrete it your sleep may be affected at times. Taking occasional sleeping pills whilst you detoxify might be preferable to nights of sleeplessness, or you could try reducing your detoxification programme.
- If you experience night sweats, vivid dreams or feel woken suddenly in the early hours of the morning, it may be because your blood sugar levels are crashing. A late-night snack of nuts and/or seeds may stave off hypoglycaemia during the night. If you wake and feel the need to eat, then you either have an addiction (intolerance) or hypoglycaemia. Please refer to advice in chapter 14.
- Whilst there are other aids such as hypnosis CDs that might be of benefit, the problem is actually biochemical so some of these may prove to be of limited value, but may be worth trying. Try all the above and the supplements detailed in chapter 17 before resorting to the pharmaceutical solutions listed below.

Pharmaceuticals for Insomnia

- Various products containing the hormone melatonin are freely available for use in the USA.
- Long-acting sedating antihistamines such as Nytol induce drowsiness and may also help, but should only be taken at the beginning of the night because of their prolonged action.
- Sedating antidepressants such as amitriptyline, temazepam and diazepam can help, but you can become dependent upon these drugs to sleep and

experience rebound insomnia when you stop taking them, for which reason you need to gradually reduce your dose.

Regular Detoxification Treatments
Colonic Hydrotherapy

The naturopathic view is that all disease starts in the bowel and so this is the logical place to begin treatment for any ailment. If the diet is not sufficiently fibrous or the processes of digestion are compromised, then over time faecal matter becomes impacted with dried mucous in the bowel wall. This prevents the absorption of nutrients and water, serves as a breeding ground for yeasts and parasites, acts as an internal 'plaster cast' preventing effective peristalsis, and the toxins produced by this biomass are absorbed and routed *directly to the liver* in the portal vein. The liver may struggle to process these endogenous toxins in addition to all the exogenous toxins it is being assaulted by and this process is known as 'auto-toxaemia' or 'auto-intoxification'. The deposits may be responsible for the symptoms of constipation because the bowel contents cannot effectively be propelled along and, paradoxically, also for diarrhoea because the deposits prevent water being absorbed from the faecal waste. Finally, most of the toxins that are currently making you ill will be processed by the liver and excreted as bile and if not rapidly expelled can be reabsorbed, retoxifying the body.

No other therapeutic approach will have much of an impact as long as the contents of your colon continue to leach into your body, so an essential first step to recovery is to remove these deposits – and absolutely everyone has them by mid-life. For this reason it is a good idea to begin all treatment with an initial course of several sessions of colonic hydrotherapy with a suitably qualified practitioner. This treatment seeks to flush out deposits from the colon using water under gentle pressure and may or may not also involve taking supplements to assist the process. Obviously access to the colon is initially required, but other than that treatment is not usually unpleasant and all the waste is carried away in a closed system. Between two and four maintenance visits per year thereafter will maintain your colon in good order. You may also wish to have more sessions if you are going through a period of intense detoxification or if you are experiencing unpleasant detoxification symptoms as this will remove the toxins being excreted into the intestine and prevent reabsorption. Iridologists regard a brown 'halo' around the pupil of the eye as an indication of the extent of deposits in the colon and with effective treatment you will also notice this diminish.

Therapeutic Baths

Baths are a good way of drawing toxins out of the body because the skin is one of the routes of excretion and has a large surface area. Conversely, for the same reason therapeutic baths are a good medium for absorbing nutrients such as magnesium.

Magnetic Clay Baths

It is possible to purchase magnetic bentonite clays combined with herbal formulations that are specific to various metals and these can be used as foot baths or in the bath. If you are intending to use these clays in bath water, you may also need to order a drain filter to prevent your drains becoming blocked; alternatively, the mixture can be emptied into a toilet.

Epsom Salt Baths

A couple of cupfuls of Epsom salts added to hot bath water act as a great source of magnesium that can be absorbed directly through the skin into the body. Soak in the bath until the water starts to cool and repeat this three times a week if possible. In addition to providing magnesium, the Epsom salts draw toxins from the body, reduce swelling, relax muscles and sedate the nervous system.

Gall Bladder and Liver Flushes

Not to be confused with a liver cleanse intended to aid regeneration of the liver, flushes are designed to remove the fatty and calcified stones that form in the *duct system* of the liver (known as the biliary tree) and the gall bladder. Gallstones are accretions of cholesterol that have usually crystallized around a fragment of parasite or Candida and the average adult is estimated to have *two to three thousand*. Some of these stones may be quite small (lentil-sized), but some may be very large indeed (several centimetres) and they individually and/or collectively can obstruct or partially obstruct the bile ducts. As this occurs elimination of fat-soluble toxins such as toxic metals via the bile is compromised and as less bile is synthesized, blood cholesterol levels rise. Those with FRS may be particularly prone to stone formation due to hypothyroidism causing stagnation of the bile and/or the liver phase II methylation detoxification pathway becoming overloaded. This technique is definitely not for the faint-hearted, but it is a cheap and effective way to improve digestion, treat allergies, eliminate shoulder, upper arm and upper back pain, lower cholesterol levels and increase energy and well-being. It is advisable to have cleansed the colon, to have cleared any parasites and to have completed your amalgam replacement before doing a liver flush unless under the guidance of a natural health professional. As someone who has removed over 4,000 gall and liver stones over 40 of these flushes, I can assure you that it is not quite as daunting in practice as it may first appear in principle. Whilst not the most pleasant 24 hours you are ever likely to experience, the whole process is surprisingly safe for people of all ages and debilities.

You will need to set aside a quiet evening and the following morning or day in order to do the flush. Please refer to figure 22 for details of the procedure and try to ensure that your timing does not deviate by more than 15 minutes from the times specified.

Figure 22: The gall bladder and liver flush schedule

Schedule	Instructions	Reason
Week prior **During the day**	Sip one litre of apple juice a day over the course of a week	The apple juice softens the stones.
Day 1 **Breakfast**	Take only those medicines or supplements that you cannot live without. Eat a no-fat breakfast, e.g. porridge made with water.	The no-fat meals mean that the gall bladder fills with bile but does not empty.
Lunch	Eat a no-fat lunch, e.g. baked potato and chopped vegetables or baked beans.	
2–6pm	Do not eat or drink anything other than water.	
6pm	Mix 3 tablespoons of Epsom salts with 4 cups of water and drink *1 cup*. Refrigerate for taste.	The Epsom salts drinks act as a laxative and relax all the valves involved. The laxative effects may be experienced later on day 1, during the night or the next day so make sure you are near a toilet.
8pm	Drink another cup of Epsom salts.	
10pm	Get ready for bed first and then shake the juice of half a reasonably sized grapefruit with an equivalent amount of olive oil in a container, drink and lie down on your back *immediately*.	The olive oil mixture causes the gall bladder and ducts in the liver to contract expelling stones. You may have some sense of what is happening, but it is not usually uncomfortable.
Day 2 **On waking**	You can get washed and dressed first and then drink the third cup of Epsom salts and *lie down*.	These Epsom salts drinks flush the stones that have been expelled into the intestine out. The stones are different colours, but mostly green and float because they are made of fat. It is worth keeping a running total of the number of stones you have removed.
2 hours later	Optional: Drink the last cup of Epsom salts and *lie down*.	
Lunch	Eat a light lunch – avoid meat and alcohol for the rest of the day.	Congratulations – you have just removed some of your gall stones without surgery.

After the first few flushes, drinking apple juice prior to the flush and the second lot of Epsom salts on day two may be surplus to requirements. You will also need to repeat the flush many times for best effect, but try and leave at least two weeks between flushes to allow stones to move down the duct system.

Pharmaceutical Drugs

If you are currently regularly taking either over-the-counter or prescription medication look at the list of side effects and consider the possibility that these drugs might be causing some or all of your symptoms. *All* pharmaceuticals are toxic and have unwanted side effects but statins, beta blockers, diuretics and antidepressants are particularly implicated in causing FRS-type symptoms. If you think one or more of your medications could be causing your symptoms discuss this with your doctor who may be willing to prescribe an alternative or supervise your efforts to reduce your dose. You may need to recruit the services of someone experienced in naturopathic principles to help support your body *before* trying to reduce the number or amount of pharmaceuticals that you take.

Paracetamol/Acetominophen

Paracetamol or Acetominophen is an analgesic which is included in many over-the-counter painkillers and various cold and flu medications. It is particularly toxic to the liver and can cause irreversible damage within or above the therapeutic dose and is the *most common cause of liver failure*. Consider using alternatives if you regularly take paracetamol-containing pharmaceuticals.

The Contraceptive Pill and HRT

The contraceptive pill, HRT, various hormone-releasing implants and coils, and depot (slow-releasing) injections are all forms of steroids. All these products disrupt the feedback mechanisms of the endocrine system and it is *almost impossible* to recover your health whilst continuing to supplement with synthetic sex hormones. Progesterone is known as the pregnancy hormone (pro-gestation) because it serves the very important function of suppressing your immune system by about 50 per cent during pregnancy so that it will not attack the 'foreign' proteins of the baby which originate from the father. Unfortunately, supplementing progesterone has devastating effects on the immune system and turns off your own innate sex hormone production which can take many months or years to recover. Taking sex hormones has also been shown to increase the incidence of breast and cervical cancer, to interfere with trace element and B vitamin metabolism and to cause mental disturbance. Obviously, if taken as a contraceptive, you need to use alternative means of birth control if discontinuing these products.

Antacids

Antacids taken for indigestion or what is perceived to be an 'acid' stomach are also worthy of a special mention in this category. The underlying problem is usually that the stomach is actually *low in acid* and this means that food is retained and churned in the stomach and only permitted to progress when sufficiently acidic. Antacids abort this process and improperly digested food is allowed to pass onwards into the alimentary tract with grave effects on the bowel flora. Endogenous production of stomach acid can also cease *within three days* of taking antacids meaning that once started, they can then become very hard to discontinue. Antacids are also thought to promote the development of allergies by preventing termination of the immune response. Finally, using laxatives is also particularly damaging since these work by irritating and sloughing the lining of the intestines.

Recreational Drugs

The use of recreational drugs can both precipitate and perpetuate the symptoms of FRS. All mood-altering substances attach to receptor sites intended for your own feel-good hormones and induce reactions within the cell. The body responds to this over-stimulation by reducing the number of receptors present in the cell membrane which means that you feel worse than before when you don't take the drug and you need more and more of it to get the same kick. If you have been using recreational drugs and you want to recover, you have to stop using drugs completely. Ask your doctor about the support that is available to help you quit if you feel you need it.

A Change of Mind

> The person who takes medicine must recover twice, once from the disease and once from the medicine.

Dr William Osler

From now on, aim to support your body using natural products and methods and to avoid pharmaceuticals wherever possible. Try to avoid the temptation to suppress your body's efforts to recover its equilibrium, no matter how unwelcome the symptoms may be. The body is far, far wiser than we will ever be and it is trying to manage an overwhelming situation in the best way possible. Some of the symptoms of detoxification can be extremely unpleasant, but take heart from the fact that by the time this occurs, your efforts to recover your health are working and your body is getting stronger and expelling the toxins that have been making you so ill. Allopathic medicine has defined many of the symptoms of detoxification such as a fever or a rash as 'disease' and medicates to eradicate the symptom. However, in suppressing the body's own innate intelligence, we thwart its efforts to detoxify and in the process, drive toxins deeper into the tissues, resulting in more and more profound illness further down the line.

Pacing

Many who ultimately end up with FRS have been living on adrenaline for years and their illness is often a huge source of frustration to them as it forces a much slower pace of life upon them. Usually any premature attempts to revert to their old ways are met with some kind of undeniable sign. Whereas – like the tortoise and the hare – accepting that your ability is compromised and just keeping a steady pace ultimately gets you to your destination faster. Previously you had, let us say, 100 'energy units' to spend each day, and now you may find that you effectively only have 10 or 20 – so spend them wisely. This means that you need to prioritize everything in your life and then only address those things that are most important to *you*. Don't allow what others think or what you imagine others might think to determine your agenda.

One of the distinctions worth making is the difference between important and urgent tasks. Urgent things demand your attention *now* whereas important things like making time to exercise or cook nutritious meals often get relegated to second place but need to be prioritized. Consider recruiting someone to do any jobs such as ironing, cleaning or gardening that can be delegated and then accept that others may either not do the job in the way you would like or to the standards you would like. You may need to downgrade your standards of housework and make life easier for yourself by buying bedding and clothing that do not need ironing and a dishwasher if you don't have one. Try to standardize your weekly shopping and cooking so you don't have to think, and arrange for regular deliveries of staple supermarket items over the Internet if possible.

Exercise

We are designed to be active and move, and we function best when we do. Exercise builds muscle and bone density, a strong heart and lungs, gets lymph pumping, aids digestion, helps to regulate mood and sleep, maintains posture and also mobilizes toxins out of storage and prevents their re-deposition. If you are very unwell it may be the last thing you feel like doing, but no exercise at all is going to see you on a slippery slope to infirmity. Forget what you used to be able to do and focus on incorporating even a little light exercise into your day, ideally outdoors. It is important that you listen to your body and that you like the exercise – or can learn to like the exercise – or you will not maintain it for any meaningful length of time. Try a gentle walk in nature, gardening, playing with your kids, swimming or stretching, cycling or a gentle exercise class. Rebounding is particularly effective for promoting circulation of stagnating lymph, is kind to painful joints and can be done indoors. If you are so weak that even light exercise seems impossible (and even if you are not) you might want to consider trying a chi exerciser. This is a shoe-box-sized electrical device that you place your ankles in whilst lying down and it generates chi (life-force energy) and promotes lymphatic circulation by rocking your legs. You may also wish to consider wearing sandals or trainers for some of the day which have been developed to emulate the more natural conditions that we evolved to walk in. Developed after studying the beautiful posture of the Masai tribesmen, Masai Barefoot Technology (MBT) trainers certainly deploy different muscles and may provide some relief of the chronic pain and stiffness so many FRS sufferers experience. Some people with FRS may find that regular physical therapy such as physiotherapy, chiropractic, osteopathy or massage may help to alleviate their more physical symptoms too. The Perrin technique was specifically created to address the physical symptoms of CFS and involves manual stimulation of the lymph and cerebrospinal fluid along with other techniques and may prove helpful. Some may also find a one-off treatment to align the atlas bone (the pivoting vertebra on which the skull articulates with the spine) known as an Atlas Profilax treatment to be beneficial. The atlas bone is displaced in most people, thus applying pressure to the spinal cord and causing back, head and neck problems. Treatment involves a somewhat vigorous mechanical massage of the back of the neck to allow the atlas bone to resume its rightful position and results in relief of back pain and other symptoms for many.

Chlorinated Water

The chlorine absorbed during an average shower is estimated to be *ten times* the amount that you would consume if you drank chlorinated water all day. If possible, have a filter fitted on your domestic water supply. Alternatively, baths can be drawn hot and left to cool for a while which allows much of the chlorine to evaporate and shower heads that filter the water are also available and can be bought online.

Piercings and Tattoos

Any piercings will provide a potential source of metal toxicity and interfere with energy flows within the body, but those in the midline of the body (affecting the central reservoir meridian) and the outer eyebrow (the endocrine system meridian) are particularly detrimental. Such piercings should be removed and either discarded or, at the very least, replaced with plastic for the majority of the time.

The inks used in tattooing are primarily metal salts with the red ink being mercury-based, although some are plastics or vegetable dyes. There is no requirement on the manufacturers to disclose the contents of the inks, but all are obviously foreign substances and become permanent because they disable the immune cells that appear at the scene to defend the body from attack.

Chapter 17
Supplementation

> The human body heals itself and nutrition provides the
> resources to accomplish the task.
>
> **Dr Roger Williams**

We now know that detoxification is an entirely nutrient dependent process and given the nutrient deficient state of our foods and the extent of the toxic assault on our systems, supplementation is an essential part of any detoxification programme. The information presented in this chapter is not intended to replace the advice of a suitably qualified practitioner, but to act as a framework for those who cannot find or cannot afford such help. The recommendations are necessarily a 'one size fits all' programme which ideally require modifying to your unique and dynamic requirements as your needs change throughout treatment.

The Time Scale for Recovery

Typically, by the time you are suffering from FRS and have initiated treatment you will be trying to reverse decades of chronic mercury and toxin exposure. So be patient, it took you a long time to become so sick and you need to understand that it is going to take you quite a long time to get better. Unlike pharmaceuticals, most supplements exert a gentle supportive influence over a period of months and their beneficial effects may not be obvious to you for some time. Indeed, your health may improve so gradually that you may quickly forget how ill you were. For this reason, it is worth jotting down a dated list of symptoms and rating them for severity and then monitoring your progress in this way every few months. As your body becomes stronger and your organs of detoxification receive the support they need, your healing will gather pace. However, there is an upper limit to what the body can detoxify at any given time and there is definitely a limit to what you may be prepared to tolerate as you detoxify.

Attempts to accelerate treatment are often met with a reminder of just how noxious the toxins you are attempting to detoxify are and how much you need to be mindful of the processes involved.

Sickness comes on horseback but departs on foot.

To give you an idea of the magnitude of what needs to occur, please refer to figure 23 which shows a very simplified version of just a few of the various body compartments that the body needs to detoxify. The body is constantly prioritizing which compartment to detoxify given the nutrients available at any particular moment, and be assured that whilst its priorities may not be the same as yours, it is working in your highest

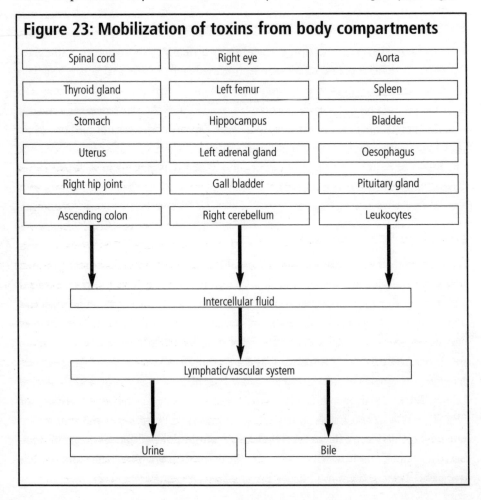

Figure 23: Mobilization of toxins from body compartments

Spinal cord	Right eye	Aorta
Thyroid gland	Left femur	Spleen
Stomach	Hippocampus	Bladder
Uterus	Left adrenal gland	Oesophagus
Right hip joint	Gall bladder	Pituitary gland
Ascending colon	Right cerebellum	Leukocytes

Intercellular fluid

Lymphatic/vascular system

Urine

Bile

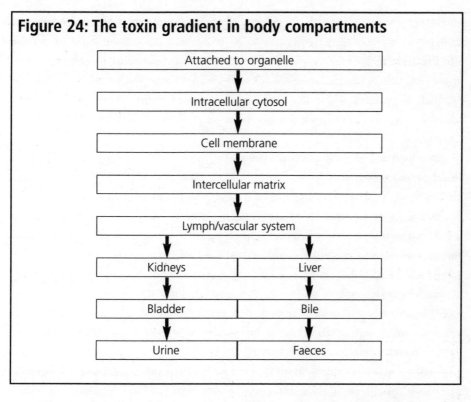

Figure 24: The toxin gradient in body compartments

interests at all times and addressing the most life-threatening issues first. Toxins will be mobilized from the extracellular space first and then progressively from the intracellular cytosol and organelles and this creates a toxin gradient that encourages the deeper tissues to detoxify as shown in figure 24. A rough guide to the likely duration of treatment might be that for every year of determined detoxification you may be able to clear approximately a decade of accumulated toxins. The toxins will be stripped away in 'layers', so if you have any symptoms of very long standing (that possibly started in childhood), these will necessarily take longer to resolve than any symptoms that appeared later in life. So the treatment programme is for the long haul. As mentioned previously, once the detoxification starts in earnest, you may experience some (possibly very) unpleasant symptoms and chapter 19 explores this subject in detail.

About Supplements

There is an old saying that 'You get what you pay for and pay for what you get' and this is as true of supplements as of anything else. The quality of supplements that you buy is crucial and high quality will not be cheap. The cheaper products may contain nutrients that are not in their active form, that are less pure or even contaminated or contain so little active ingredient as to be worthless. These products may not be effective and this obviously represents a waste of money and effort, but perhaps more importantly steals more of your life and may crush your hopes of a recovery. Specific products are named where necessary, but an independent retailer will be able to advise you and you can order either online or over the telephone from most reputable companies.

If you have not taken supplements before, the amounts involved may seem excessive. However, remember that you are trying to eliminate one of the most potent toxins known to man from 100 trillion cells. It is also worth mentioning that the recommended daily allowances (RDA) of various nutrients vary enormously from one country to another and have been set at levels below which *deficiency symptoms* appear and bear no relation to optimal health. The amount of nutrients required will also vary greatly according to such factors as age, weight, gender and activity and so any recommendations are necessarily an average and most seriously ill people may require many multiples of the recommended amount of some nutrients. Any excess of water-soluble vitamins will be excreted in the urine, but you do need to be careful not to exceed the RDA of the fat-soluble vitamin A in particular.

If you are new to supplementation or if your health is extremely compromised and you know that you are likely to react poorly, *start gently with very low doses, introducing one supplement at a time.* If your digestion is seriously compromised you may also not be digesting or absorbing much of what you do take and using the digestive enzymes suggested or taking liquid or tincture forms may help with this. Also, because everyone is different, not all supplements agree with all people, so you may need to modify any recommendations to your unique biochemistry. There is almost no point starting the natural recovery plan if you are only likely to take one or two pots of each supplement or be erratic about supplementing. Ultimately, what counts is being consistent over time and for this reason it is worth buying 'pill minder' boxes and having a routine where you fill them every weekend. Some of these have removable strips which makes taking your supplements with you when you go out or to work easier and therefore more likely to occur. It is also worth establishing a convenient way of buying supplements by ordering online or over the telephone.

When it comes to determining which supplements are required and in what quantities, learning to dowse or muscle test will prove invaluable. Please refer to the Appendix for more details.

The Suggested Supplement Protocol

The suggested overall approach to supplementation is shown in figure 25 and involves primarily detoxifying via the bile and intestines. This is considered to be safer than attempting to detoxify via the urine. This is because the delicate structures in the kidneys cannot be replaced, whereas the intestinal lining is regenerated every few days. This method, however, does mean that the bowel flora is damaged and that diarrhoea or at least soft bowel movements may occur at times during the detoxification. The use of probiotics throughout the detoxification has not been specified because there is some concern that they contribute to the methylation of inorganic mercury. If you experience loose bowel movements, you may want to either test probiotics as suggested in the Appendix or experiment for yourself and see whether you feel better or worse for including them in the protocol and then act appropriately.

The approach to detoxification suggested here will work in the majority of cases *irrespective* of which particular toxic metals or microbes you may have been affected by. As the body is assisted to detoxify and excrete the toxic metals, various viruses and bacteria that have been stored in the cells but never fully eliminated will become active and an antimicrobial supplement (Samento tincture) is recommended to resolve this. There are usually several latent viruses or bacteria in total and these will surface one at a time throughout the detoxification and require eliminating as they appear. As toxicity is addressed, many of the other secondary issues, such as candidal or parasitic

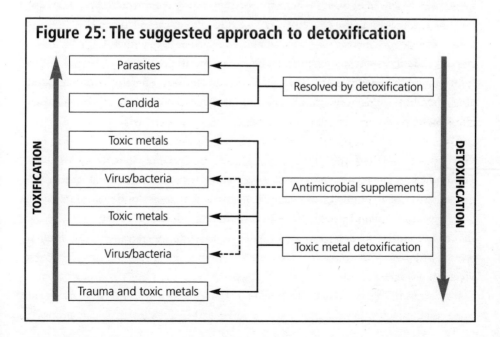

Figure 25: The suggested approach to detoxification

Figure 26: Suggested protocol

Phase	Time scale
Initial	
Colon cleanse	Weeks 1–4
Detoxification	
Pre-amalgam removal	Several months < 2 years
Amalgam removal	Weeks/months
Post-amalgam removal*	Several months < 2 years
Repair	
Repair and special support	Several months
Maintenance	Lifetime

*If you cannot afford to, or do not intend to have your amalgam fillings replaced, you can proceed to post-amalgam removal detoxification protocol shown in figures 38 and 39 after a few months or when you feel well enough.

infections, will be resolved by the body with little or no further intervention as the general milieu and the immune system improve. In order to enjoy complete restoration of health, every last little bit of toxic metal and every microbe requires removal. Using this technique allows you to overcome rather than manage your FRS. The first half of the body burden of toxic metals are often detoxified and excreted relatively rapidly with the remaining half being released more slowly and possibly requiring the input of a professional experienced in these matters. Some issues are often resolved relatively early on in treatment including the overgrowth of Candida, however neurological symptoms, poor memory and introversion, for instance, may take longer to rectify.

The suggested protocol is shown in figure 26 and involves various phases lasting from a month to many months. To avoid confusion and keep the information targeted, only a handful of the many hundreds of supplements that might be of benefit to the FRS sufferer have been selected.

Important Considerations

This protocol is presented as a framework only and is not intended to replace the advice of a suitably qualified practitioner. Please also note that your blood cholesterol levels may *temporarily increase* while detoxifying mercury. Women of reproductive age should not undertake any form of detoxification *if they are either pregnant, likely to become pregnant or are nursing*. However, detoxifying *before* any attempt to become pregnant will help to prevent toxins being passed to your baby both in your womb and in your breast milk. This advice is intended for adults and detoxification of children and babies is approached in a different manner and is a specialist subject. The quantities of supplements suggested relate to most normal-weight adults, but should be modified for both the significantly under- or overweight. Please also read the notes pertaining to each supplement and particularly the special cautions that apply to the use of Samento and Cilantro tinctures.

Initial Phase

The suggested protocol starts with cleansing the colon first for four weeks and this is very necessary to prepare for efficient elimination and should not be omitted in your haste to get started. You can skip this phase if you have opted for a course of colonic hydrotherapy instead.

Colon Cleanse

The goals of this phase of treatment are to remove the deposits from the bowel walls that enable the overgrowth of fungi and parasites and prevent the absorption of nutrients and water. This also removes a major source of auto-toxicity, thus relieving the ongoing burden on the liver. When free of their deposits the bowel walls can also propel matter along more efficiently, enabling the rapid removal of toxic bile with little opportunity afforded for reabsorption. Although the colon cleanse should not be followed for more than four weeks at a time, you may choose to repeat this phase of treatment every six months or so. Please refer to figure 27 for details and to figure 28 for a summary.

Optional Liver Cleanse

Liver detoxification is always seriously compromised in all chronic illnesses and you may wish to do an initial liver cleanse after the colon cleanse and periodically throughout treatment. Products such as Metagenic's Ultraclear Plus pH and Thorne's Mediclear are available through your natural health practitioner and have been specifically formulated to boost liver detoxification in those whose health is seriously compromised. They are powders that are made up into drinks and whilst they can be of great benefit, if you are very fragile you will need to start *extremely tentatively* and increase the dose *very gradually*. However, if you find that you can tolerate these products or can work up to a reasonable dose, an occasional intensive week or few weeks of use every few months will accelerate treatment. Small daily doses can also be used throughout detoxification or for maintenance.

Figure 27: Initial colon cleanse

Supplement	**Bentonite and psyllium husk shakes (B & P shakes)**
	Bentonite (Montmorillonite) clay is a special type of clay which can be bought as a powder or liquid (which is easier to mix). It can be ordered over the Internet.
Suggested dose	One tablespoon of liquid bentonite clay can be added to a teaspoon of psyllium husks, mixed with water or juice and drunk immediately (use a plastic spoon to mix). Start slowly with 1 shake a day and build to 3 shakes a day. To prevent constipation it is very important that you drink plenty of water and drink at least one glass of water after each shake.
Benefits	Bentonite clay has special magnetic properties that pull toxins (especially toxic metals) out through the intestine walls and also trap and remove Candida. The psyllium husks are absorptive and have the effect of regulating bowel function.
Cautions	Because of the magnetic properties of the bentonite clay, you could (theoretically at least) become nutrient deficient if you continued with this programme for more than a month. For this reason the shakes should also be taken at least one hour away from food, supplements or medication. If you are taking life-sustaining medication or have high blood pressure, consult your doctor first. Note that your faeces might smell quite offensive whilst you are following this regime and may look odd as old faecal deposits are expelled.

Supplement	**Multimineral/multivitamin**
	A good quality multimineral/multivitamin tailored for you (male/female) and your current circumstances (over/under 40 for men and pre/postmenopausal for women). This should be copper and iron free because these minerals can promote production of free radicals.
Suggested dose	Take the maximum amount suggested by the manufacturer, dividing the dose between the breakfast and evening meal.
Benefits	Vitamins and minerals are essential to every reaction that takes place within the body, support the immune system and are necessary for normal function and growth. Minerals in particular are required in relatively large quantities by the endocrine system and facilitate detoxification in general and metal detoxification in particular. Most FRS sufferers require the B vitamins which aid release of energy from food.
Cautions	Do not exceed 750mcg of vitamin A per day as retinol if you are pregnant or likely to become pregnant.
	Seek advice if you are taking anticoagulant medication.
	Products containing B vitamins may colour the urine. This is perfectly normal and nothing to be concerned about although increasing quantities of water drunk will dilute the urine.

Supplement	**Vitamin C**
	1g vitamin C tablets (buffered, timed release and/or combined with bioflavonoids) or as an ascorbate drink. Magnesium deficiency is often found in FRS, so a product containing magnesium ascorbate will supply both magnesium and vitamin C.
Suggested dose	4g/day in divided doses.
Benefits	Vitamin C is required in quite high doses as it is protective against many toxins (particularly toxic metals) and converts fat-soluble methyl mercury into the water-soluble form so that it can be mobilized and excreted. Vitamin C is also essential for tissue repair, formation of red blood cells and immunity, supportive of adrenal gland function, inhibitory of allergic reactions, and is a powerful antioxidant for the water-soluble component of the body acting in concert with vitamin E in the fat-soluble compartment. Many FRS sufferers may also be vitamin C deficient through long-term use of either the contraceptive pill or aspirin.
Cautions	Check with your doctor if you have kidney stones or haemachromatosis and start gently if you have gout.
	High doses of vitamin C *may interfere with the effectiveness of the contraceptive pill* (additional contraception may be required) and should not be taken at the same time of day.
	Very high doses of vitamin C may cause loose bowel movements, and doses should be reduced if this occurs.

Figure 27: cont.

Supplement **Fish oils/flax seed oil**

Aim for 240–300mg EPA/160–200mg DHA per serving. Only buy products that are guaranteed free of heavy metals and organic contaminants. If vegetarian or vegan take generous amounts of flax seed oil, but most mercury-toxic individuals have difficulty converting this to EPA which is the form that is highly beneficial to the nervous system.

Suggested dose 500 mg fish oils three times a day. If vegetarian or vegan take the maximum dose of flax seed oil recommended by the manufacturer.

Benefits Essential fatty acids are involved in the production of energy and the transport of oxygen; are anti-inflammatory; are involved in repair and maintenance of cell structure; protect the nervous system against viral infection; decrease inflammation in joints and muscles; improve dry skin; normalize immune response and 'autoimmunity'; are greatly beneficial to the cardiovascular system; enhance brain function and relieve depression; help to prevent 'leaky gut'; aid treatment of food allergies; help to maintain gut flora; aid glandular secretions and increase levels of HDL (good) cholesterol and decrease levels of LDL (bad) cholesterol.

Cautions Do not use if you are a haemophiliac or epileptic and consult your doctor if you are taking anticoagulant medication.
Fish oils should not have an aftertaste or smell fishy – if they do they have oxidised. Keep supplements containing oils in the fridge where possible and consume before the 'use by' date.

Supplement **Digestive enzymes**

Try either a broad-spectrum digestive enzyme formulation including bile and/or pepsin and betaine hydrochloride which is intended to replace stomach acid and initiate the proper digestion of proteins. If vegan or vegetarian plant digestive enzyme formulations are available.

Suggested dose Take pepsin and betaine hydrochloride either with protein meals only or with every meal and/or take a broad spectrum digestive enzyme with every meal (depending upon how compromised your digestion is).

Benefits All FRS sufferers have compromised production of digestive enzymes, particularly in the stomach. Proper breakdown of foodstuffs will help to normalize bowel flora, minimize food intolerances and allergies, and provide the nutrients required for tissue repair and proper functioning of the immune system.

Cautions Do not take if you have any history of ulcerative conditions of the alimentary tract including gastritis. If you feel discomfort after taking the product either reduce the dose or discontinue. Swallow tablets whole shortly before eating.

Figure 28: Summary of initial colon cleanse

Supplement	Breakfast	Mid-morning	Lunch	Mid-afternoon	Evening meal	Late evening
B & P shakes	—	1 shake	—	1 shake	—	1 shake
Multimineral/vitamin	1–2 caps	—	—	—	1–2 caps	—
Vitamin C	2g	—	1g	—	1g	—
Fish oils/flax seed oil	2–3 caps	—	2–3 caps	—	2–3 caps	—
Digestive enzymes	(1 tab)	—	1–2 tabs	—	1–2 tabs	—

Detoxification Phase
Pre-Amalgam Removal

The supplement protocol outlined in figure 29 and summarized in figure 30 may need to be followed for a year or more. The aim of this phase of treatment is to generally reduce all the readily accessible mercury and toxin levels within the body. You are attempting to reduce the amounts of mercury in the intercellular matrix so that movement out of the cells can then be facilitated. If you have amalgam fillings, you should follow this protocol until you feel well enough to have them replaced. Rinsing after meals with Dentacare mouthwash may help to reduce mercury absorbtion into the tissues of the mouth in the interim. If you do not have amalgam fillings this part of the detoxification should be followed for a few months in order to generally decrease the accessible toxins before attempting to progress to the post-amalgam removal detoxification phase. You may or may not notice any immediate benefits of this part of treatment; however, it is a necessary precursor to the post-amalgam detoxification protocol which then seeks to draw toxins out of deep storage. Again, use your judgement and if you are very reactive, start with low doses of Chlorella and *slowly introduce the other supplements one at a time*, starting with the vitamin C and introducing the milk thistle and other supplements *gradually*. If you can only afford, or are only willing to take one supplement, then the Chlorella taken consistently over a year or two would be my choice – ideally combined with reasonable doses of vitamin C.

Additional Supplements

You may wish to include additional supplements to support specific issues either periodically or throughout your detoxification and these are detailed in the following tables. For additional support for emotional issues refer to figure 31; for support of detoxification see figure 32; for the physical symptoms of FRS see figure 33; for issues of an under-functioning immune system or fungal overgrowth see figure 34; and for endocrine support see figure 35. Additionally, if you have had occupational exposure to a particular toxin you may wish to take a product such as those formulated by Thorne Research which are toxin specific such as Formaldehyde relief, Solvent remover and Pesticide protector.

Figure 29: Pre-amalgam removal detoxification protocol

Supplement	**Multimineral/multivitamin**		
Suggested dose	Divide maximum dose between meals.		
Benefits	For details see figure 27.	Cautions	For details see figure 27.
Supplement	**Vitamin C**		
Suggested dose	1g three times a day.		
Benefits	For details see figure 27.	Cautions	For details see figure 27.
Supplement	**Fish oils/flax seed oil**		
Suggested dose	500mg fish oils three times a day.		
Benefits	For details see figure 27.	Cautions	For details see figure 27.
Supplement	**Digestive enzymes**		
Suggested dose	Taken with protein only or all meals.		
Benefits	For details see figure 27.	Cautions	For details see figure 27.
Supplement	**Psyllium husks**		
	As powder or capsules can be bought online or at most health food shops. Other products such as apple pectin and acacia can provide similar sources of fibre if required.		
Suggested dose	If powdered, a level teaspoon stirred into a glass of juice or water and drunk immediately once or twice a day. Dose capsules as suggested by the manufacturer and drink plenty of water.		
Benefits	Required to maintain regular bowel movements and prevent reabsorption of toxic bile. Acts as an 'internal broom' cleaning accumulated debris from the bowel walls.		
Cautions	Ensure that you are drinking the recommended amount of water with this product and it is a good idea to drink a glass of water after each psyllium husk drink.		
Supplement	**Selenium**		
	Some forms of selenium are derived from yeast, so if this is a particular problem for you look for a yeast-free form of selenium.		
Suggested dose	1 x 200mcg capsule twice a day.		
Benefits	Binds to mercury; is a natural antioxidant; protects the brain and kidneys; prevents viruses from reproducing; essential for thyroid gland function; is involved in immunity; is anti-fungal and antibacterial; aids retention of magnesium.		
Cautions	If sensitive to petrochemicals start slowly and gently increase dose. Ideally, you should leave two hours between taking selenium and vitamin C. As selenium is antifungal, antibacterial and antiviral it may produce symptoms of die-off or the Herxheimer reaction.		
Supplement	**Vitamin E**		
	Vitamin E consists of eight chemicals known as tocopherols and tocotrienols. Avoid the synthetic 'dl' forms – look for d-alpha tocopherol and mixed tocopherols 120IU (80mg).		
Suggested dose	1 capsule 120IU/80mg mixed tocopherols three times a day.		
Benefits	Protects red blood cells; is required for proper cell membrane function; prevents the formation of LDL (bad) cholesterol; aids cellular respiration increasing muscle endurance and stamina; absorbed into the lymph it concentrates in the fatty tissues where it acts as a powerful antioxidant that recycles vitamin C; has antiviral properties and helps to repair viral damage.		
Cautions	Start slowly. Vitamin E can interfere with iron metabolism in high doses. Consult your doctor if taking anti-coagulant medication or antifungal medication for ringworm.		
Supplement	**Milk thistle**		
	Also known as Silymarin or Silybum marianum. Is often complexed with other herbs known to support liver function such as dandelion, artichoke or turmeric.		
Suggested dose	1 capsule containing approximately 200mg milk thistle three times a day.		
Benefits	Milk thistle contains constituents that enhance liver function by up to a third whilst providing powerful antioxidant protection. Milk thistle also promotes the detoxification of mercury; aids tissue regeneration by enhancing the rate of protein synthesis in the liver and protects and aids regeneration of the kidneys.		
Cautions	Not recommended for those with obstructed bile ducts or gallstones. If taking medication, seek professional advice.		

continued on next page

Figure 29: cont.

Supplement	**Chlorella pyrenoidosa**
	Chlorella is a single-celled, fresh water algae that is rich in protein, vitamins, minerals, Chlorella growth factor and other beneficial substances. It has developed numerous protective mechanisms over millennia for binding toxins in general and toxic metals in particular. It is widely used in Asia from where most supplements originate. There are two forms: Chlorella pyrenoidosa which has superior toxin absorbing qualities, but which is less digestible and Chlorella vulgaris which is more digestible, but has reduced toxin absorption. Ensure purity is certified as some products may not have been grown in pure water environments and as a result may have reduced toxin absorption capacity.
Suggested dose	3 x 500mg tablets three times a day before meals.
Benefits	Chlorella has developed at least 20 different mechanisms by which it binds toxins – particularly toxic metals in the soft tissues and colon. It also aids detoxification; is a super nutrient with a high protein, mineral and vitamin content that is ideal for vegetarians; has antiviral actions; increases the glutathione available for mercury detoxification; normalizes insulin resistance; enhances the immune system; restores healthy bowel flora; bulks the faeces and alkalinizes the body.
Cautions	May colour the urine and faeces. If Chlorella pyrenoidosa causes loose bowel movements reduce dose or switch to the more digestible Chlorella vulgaris form. Some people (particularly those with high cysteine levels) may find taking Chlorella problematic, in which case use an alternative metal-detoxifying agent (see figures 32 and 40). Chlorella itself is really a very safe supplement, however sometimes the body may 'confuse' it with the toxins that it is escorting out of the body and this can promote some sort of reaction. If this occurs either: switch to Chlorella vulgaris, take a break for a few weeks or use an alternative. Most reactions whilst taking Chlorella are not likely to be to the Chlorella itself but may highlight other sources of toxins which require elimination such as body care products or additives in the diet.

Supplement	**Samento tincture**
	Samento is a rare form of Cat's Claw (Uncaria tomentosa) – a medicinal rainforest plant from Peru. The herb contains alkaloids known as POAs and TOAs, and you need to find a product that is TOA free (such as Nutramedix' Samento tincture) because this component inhibits the actions of the medicinal POAs. Tinctures are able to enter all body compartments, whereas supplements taken in capsule form tend to be confined to the intestines.
Suggested dose	Samento tincture can produce potent Herxheimer reactions, for which reason when first starting to take this supplement take 2 drops twice a day and increase by a drop at each dose every second or third day until you have reached the dosage of about 10 drops twice a day. Once you have used one bottle of Samento tincture, you can resume at the previous dose. Can be included from the beginning or incorporated as viral-type symptoms appear.
Benefits	Samento has a broad spectrum of actions: it activates and normalizes the immune response (especially chemical sensitivity and autoimmunity); is anti-viral and prevents the expansion of virus-laden cells; it is also anti-fungal and antibacterial especially against Borrelia burgdorferi (Lyme disease); kills parasites; restores proper intestinal flora; aids repair of a 'leaky gut'; has powerful anti-inflammatory actions which aid joint pains and other inflammatory conditions; is a diuretic; aids repair of cell walls; stimulates the liver; decreases fatigue and stabilizes mood.
Cautions	Samento is an extraordinary herb and is primarily recommended for its antimicrobial actions, however it can produce an unpleasant Herxheimer reaction. It is quite expensive, so you may want to wait until viral-type symptoms appear such as swollen glands/tonsils; nasal symptoms; diarrhoea; rashes and headaches and pains before starting to take the Samento. If you start to experience a severe detoxification reaction, reduce the dose for a while and then gradually try to increase one drop at a time. Use with caution with hormonal pharmaceutical drugs (such as HRT or the contraceptive pill), if an insulin-dependent diabetic or when having vaccinations.

Supplement	**Dentacare mouthwash**
	This mouthwash helps to prevent the absortion of mercury into the tissues of the mouth. Available from www.evenbetternow.com.
Suggested dose	Rinsing after each meal is advised.

Figure 30: Summary of pre-amalgam removal detoxification protocol

Supplement	Breakfast	Lunch	Evening meal
Multimineral/vitamin	1–2 caps	—	1–2 caps
Vitamin C	1g*	1g*	1g*
Fish oils/flax seed oil	2–3 caps	2–3 caps	2–3 caps
Digestive enzymes	(1–2 tabs)	1–2 tabs	1–2 tabs
Psyllium husks	1 tsp	—	1 tsp
Selenium	1 cap	—	1 cap
Vitamin E	1 cap	1 cap	1 cap
Milk thistle	1 cap	1 cap	1 cap
Chlorella pyrenoidosa	3 tabs	3 tabs	3 tabs
Samento tincture	10 drops†	—	10 drops†
Dentacare mouthwash	Rinse	Rinse	Rinse

*Best taken away from the Chlorella
† See dosing guidelines in figure 29

Figure 31: Additional supplements for emotional support

Insomnia	Benefits	Cautions
5-hydroxy-tryptophan (5-HTP) Suggested dose: 50–100mg 3 times a day or 2 capsules on a sleepless night.	5-HTP is converted in the body into serotonin and ultimately melatonin, regulating sleep and elevating mood if depressed.	Consult your doctor if taking antidepressants. Very high doses may cause loose stools.
Melatonin Supplements and sublingual sprays can be obtained freely in the USA, but with restrictions in the UK. Ideally take under the supervision of a practitioner. Suggested dose: Follow manufacturer's instructions.	Melatonin induces sleep without suppressing REM (rapid eye movement or dreaming) sleep, as sedatives and other pharmaceutical aids do.	Will only be of benefit if the circulating levels of melatonin are low. Some people may get depressed using melatonin. Supplementing any hormone may affect endocrine regulation.
Herbal preparations Containing herbs such as passion flower, California poppy, kava kava or valerian. Suggested dose: Follow manufacturer's instructions.	A gentle, non-pharmaceutical aid to sleep.	See cautions on product.
St John's Wort Suggested dose: Follow manufacturer's instructions.	Helps to relieve chronic insomnia especially when accompanied by mild depression.	Can cause sun sensitivity. Consult your doctor if taking other medication. If taking the contraceptive pill additional contraception is advised.
Ultraclear or Mediclear Suggested dose: 1 to 3 scoops a day	May alleviate anxiety and if taken in the evening may help to promote sleep.	Aids the breakdown of adrenaline (epinephrine). See product for cautions. See Optional Liver Cleanse on page 185.

Figure 31: cont.

Anxiety	Benefits	Cautions
Kava kava extract		
(Standardized for kavalactone 45–70mg) **Suggested dose:** Follow manufacturer's instructions.	Calms and improves mental function; does not cause sedation at normal doses. Daily recommended dose can be taken at night to promote sleep.	Do not take with Parkinson's disease. Only use under supervision if taking benzodiazepines. May cause scaly skin if taken excessively for more than a year.
B vitamins		
Especially vitamin B1 (Thiamin) and vitamin B3 (Niacin) **Suggested dose:** Follow manufacturer's instructions.	B vitamins are essential for mental function, memory and feelings of well-being.	None known at recommended doses.

Depression	Benefits	Cautions
Adults to 50 years of age: **5-HTP** (with St John's Wort if severe) **Suggested dose:** Follow manufacturer's instructions.	See above	See above
If over 50 years of age: **Gingko Biloba** (with 5-HTP and/or St John's Wort if severe). **Suggested dose:** Follow manufacturer's instructions.	Gingko Biloba enhances cerebral circulation aiding mental function.	See cautions on product.
Gotu Kola		
Suggested dose: Follow manufacturer's instructions.	Gotu Kola aids cognitive and adrenal function, thus helping with stress and depression. It also promotes growth of healthy skin, hair and nails.	See cautions on product.

Figure 32: Additional supplements for supporting detoxification

Detoxification	Benefits	Cautions
N-Acetyl Cysteine (NAC) Suggested dose: 1 capsule containing approx. 250mg of NAC twice a day.	Mobilizes and aids excretion of metals in the urine; protects blood cells; protects the liver and aids liver detoxification; reduces mucous; is a powerful antioxidant; is anti-inflammatory; supports the immune system; crosses the blood–brain barrier and increases endogenous glutathione.	If taking medication seek professional advice. Do not take if you have cystinuria, cystinosis or high glutathione levels. Do not take more than 500mg/day. *NB: Stop taking NAC at least 5 days before a local or general anaesthetic.*
Whey protein formulations Powdered protein drinks that can be used to replace or supplement meals such as Metagenics' BioPure Protein. Avoid formulas which contain artificial sweeteners. **Suggested dose:** Follow the manufacturers' instructions.	A supplementary source of high-quality protein for general repair, maintenance and detoxification – especially for vegetarians. Whey protein is antibacterial and antiviral; is a source of glutathione; protects the liver, aids digestion and helps with weight maintenance.	Can cause insomnia, so avoid taking in the evening. May colour the urine yellow which is harmless, and drinking water will restore a more normal colour. Even those who are dairy intolerant can usually tolerate these products. Study the label for specifics.
Antioxidant formulations Many formulations contain mixtures of nutrients and carotenoids, green tea leaf extract, rutin, hesperidin, proanthocyanidins or quercetin. **Suggested dose:** Follow manufacturer's recommendations.	Counters the extensive free radical damage caused by toxicity throughout the body.	See specific cautions on product and check combined dosages of specific nutrients with other products that you may be taking.
Trace mineral formula **Suggested dose:** Follow manufacturer's recommendations.	Trace minerals are required for many enzyme systems, to prevent toxic metals re-entering the cell and for detoxification pathways.	None known if directions are followed.

Figure 32: cont.

Detoxification	Benefits	Cautions
Matrix metals		
Nanonized Chlorella and other herbs. Available from BioPure. **Suggested dose:** 2–4 sprays sub-lingually or can be used in nostrils as drops.	Aids toxic metal detoxification of the brain.	Detoxification symptoms.
Phospholipid exchange		
This is a combination of a synthetic chelator (EDTA) and phospholipids. Available from BioPure. **Suggested dose:** See manufacturer's instructions.	Aids transport across cell and blood/brain membranes; aids heart function; may reduce diarrhoea whilst detoxifiying.	See cautions on product.
Sekebal harmonie gel		
Can be obtained from specialist shops or ordered online from www.sekebal.com. **Suggested dose:** 2–3 drops of gel rubbed into the hands or feet at night, ideally over a period of 6–12 months.	This is a vibrational remedy gel that promotes detoxification from the nervous system of fungi, heavy metals and environmental toxins.	No cautions – a very gentle remedy for the old or very sick.
Rose geranium essential oil		
Suggested dose: 6 drops in bathwater or applied to the skin in a carrier oil every day.	Rose geranium oil specifically aids mercury detoxification, balances sex hormones and is antimicrobial.	None known. A gentle method of detoxifying for the elderly or infirm.

Figure 33: Additional supplements for support of physical symptoms

Joint Pain	Benefits	Cautions
Methyl Sulphonyl Methane (MSM)		
An organic form of sulphur that does not cause body odour or intestinal gas. **Dose:** 1–2 x 500mg capsules twice a day with meals.	Aids joint structure and function.	Some FRS sufferers may react to sulphur-containing products (see page 147).
Glucosamine and chondroitin		
Dose: Follow manufacturer's recommendations.	Aids with the structure and function of joints; aids removal of mercury from the intestines and joints; anti-inflammatory; relieves allergies and constipation.	None known if directions are followed.

Aching Muscles	Benefits	Cautions
Magnesium or a magnesium-based formulation		
Dose: Follow manufacturer's recommendations.	A muscle relaxant; promotes the release of energy; aids cardiovascular health and is required for calcium absorption.	See specific product for cautions.

Fatigue	Benefits	Cautions
Coenzme Q10		
Depleted by taking statins. **Dose:** Normally 1 capsule daily with food.	A potent antioxidant which concentrates in the membranes and mitochondria, aiding energy production especially in the heart, stomach and immune system; aids conversion of fat into energy so may aid weight loss.	Quite expensive.
B vitamins		
Often depleted by taking the contraceptive pill. **Dose:** One vitamin B complex tablet once or twice a day.	Aids energy production; stress response; blood sugar balance; detoxification; depression; sleep/wake cycles; the proper function of the nervous system; and cell reproduction.	Can cause insomnia, so avoid taking in the evening. May colour the urine yellow. This is harmless and drinking adequate supplies of water should restore a more normal colour.

Figure 34: Additional supplements for treatment of infections and immune support

Immune System	Benefits	Cautions
Plant Sterols Dose: Follow manufacturer's suggestions.	A modulator boosting a poor immune system and calming overactive or allergic responses; supports cardiovascular function and healthy cholesterol levels.	Do not take if you have had an organ transplant or are on immunosuppressant medication. Take under the supervision of a doctor if diabetic.
Echinacea Dose: Follow manufacturer's suggestions.	Supports the health of the immune system.	As above. Not intended for long-term use as response diminishes with time.
Astragalus Dose: Follow manufacturer's suggestions.	Antiviral; enhances the immune system.	As above. Not intended for long-term use as response diminishes with time.
Coleus Forskohlii Dose: Follow manufacturer's suggestions.	Aids energy production; counters allergic reactions; aids thyroid function; is anti-inflammatory and promotes cardiovascular function.	See product for cautions.
Antioxidant formulations A blend often including green tea, quercetin and turmeric. Dose: Follow manufacturer's suggestions.	Provide the nutrients required to counter oxidation aiding immune function and preventing ageing.	See product for cautions.

Anti-Candida	Benefits	Cautions
Anti-candidal preparations Often contain: caprylic acid; garlic; cinnamon; thyme; cloves; oregano; turmeric; cayenne; wormwood; black walnut; berberine and grapefruit seed extract. Dose: Follow manufacturer's recommendations.	Help to control candidal overgrowth and related symptoms (thrush, bloating and flatulence).	Will induce die off so start gently and increase dose slowly. Alternatively, expect to have flu-like symptoms for a few days a couple of days after starting supplementation. Pure oregano oil is an irritant and best taken in micro-encapsulated form and caprylic acid produces the most potent die-off reactions.
Probiotic powder or capsules Containing bacteria such as Lactobacillus acidophilus and/or Bifidobacterium bifidum Dose: 1–2 capsules or powder as directed with each meal.	Maintains a healthy flora in the large intestine and generally supports digestion.	Keep refrigerated and use before suggested date. Some concern that bacteria can methylate mercury, so avoid continuous use.

continued on next page

Figure 34: cont.

Anti-Candida	Benefits	Cautions
Saccharomyces boulardii A non-pathogenic yeast which supports healthy gut flora. **Dose:** Follow manufacturer's recommendations.	A probiotic which is not affected by antibiotics and can be taken at the same time; a natural source of B vitamins. Short courses aid floral balance, but unlike other probiotics, S. boulardii is not retained over time.	Not suitable for those with organ transplants or the immune-compromised.
Tea tree tincture and/or coconut oil **Dose:** Follow manufacturer's recommendations.	For topical application to fungal nails or athlete's foot.	See product for cautions.

Figure 35: Additional supplements for support of the endocrine system

Hypoadrenia/Stress	Benefits	Cautions
Siberian ginseng Sometimes complexed with liquorice. **Suggested dose:** Follow manufacturer's instructions.	Supports the adrenal glands aiding both physical and mental stress, but also has antiviral actions; boosts immune function; aids digestion; normalizes blood sugar levels.	Do not use if you have high blood pressure. Alternate with liquorice after 8 weeks.
Liquorice (Glycyrrhiza) Sometimes complexed with Siberian ginseng. **Suggested dose:** Follow manufacturer's instructions.	Supports the adrenal glands; is antiviral and anti-inflammatory; aids allergic reactions; protects the liver and has antidepressant actions.	Do not exceed suggested dose. Can raise blood pressure if taken over a long period of time – consult your doctor before use if you are hypertensive.
Ashwagandha 'Indian ginseng' **Suggested dose:** Follow manufacturer's instructions.	Immune booster; supports the adrenal glands; aids musculoskeletal pain; aids reproductive function.	Do not take if pregnant or breastfeeding. Consult your doctor if taking other medication.
Specific formulations A formulation of nutrients and herbs to support adrenal function. **Suggested dose:** Follow manufacturer's instructions.	A blend of B vitamins, minerals and herbs to support the stress response.	See cautions on product. Ensure RDA vitamin A not exceeded if taken in combination with other products.
B Vitamins Especially B5 (Pantethine) and B6 (Pyridoxone) **Suggested dose:** Follow manufacturer's instructions.	Supports adrenal gland function and aids production of energy.	None known at recommended doses.

Figure 35: cont.

Hypothyroidism	Benefits	Cautions
Specific formulations Contains a blend of nutrients required for thyroid function. Suggested dose: Follow manufacturer's instructions.	Aids thyroid function and may aid thyroxine conversion.	See cautions on product.
Coleus Forskohlii Suggested dose: Follow manufacturer's instructions.	Aids thyroid hormone conversion and circulation and inhibits allergic reactions including asthma.	See cautions on product.
Liquorice Suggested dose: Follow manufacturer's instructions.	See above	See above

Hypoglycaemia	Benefits	Cautions
Chromium Suggested dose: 100–300mcg twice a day	Supports blood sugar control and glucose uptake by the cells; may aid weight reduction.	None known at recommended doses.
Specific formulations Suggested dose: Follow manufacturer's instructions.	A blend of nutrients to support blood sugar regulation.	See cautions on product.

Figure 36: Post-amalgam removal detoxification protocol 1

Protocol as figure 29. In addition:

Supplement	Benefits	Cautions
Alpha lipoic acid (ALA) Introduce first taking every other day and build to the required dose before introducing the Cilantro tincture. **Dose:** Take no more than one capsule containing approximately 250mg of alpha lipoic acid a day for four weeks and then discontinue for two weeks before resuming.	A universal antioxidant working in both fat and water soluble compartments of the body; aids liver detoxification; regenerates other antioxidants; aids mitochondrial function and energy production; supports good neurological function and healthy blood sugar metabolism. Recommended in this context to chelate toxic metals out of fatty tissue including the brain and endocrine glands.	Can cause mineral imbalance if taken continuously, thus breaks in supplementation are recommended. Can also increase mercury in the nervous system if taken in high quantities or if easily accessible mercury is not sufficiently detoxified first. Do not exceed the manufacturer's suggested dose. *Start gently and slowly increase the dose.* Only start to introduce at least 6 weeks after the last amalgam filling is removed.
Cilantro tincture (Coriandrum sativum, Chinese parsley) Introduce after ALA dose stable with no side effects. **Dose:** Follow manufacturer's instructions with regard to dosing. A guide would be to start on a quarter of the dose and slowly build to taking 3–5 drops 2–3 times a day in warm water (ideally after all metals are removed from the mouth). Alternatively, the tincture can be rubbed into the wrists and/or ankles (to mobilize metals above and below the diaphragm respectively), the groin or other affected body parts. Take away from garlic and vitamin C if possible.	Mobilizes toxic metals out of the bone, central nervous system and fat and detaches and removes mercury from cell organelles; it also reverses DNA damage in the nucleus. Cilantro causes the gall bladder to contract secreting bile, for which reason it should ideally be taken 30 minutes after any Chlorella so that the Chlorella can absorb the toxins excreted in the bile. Note that 10–15 drops of Cilantro tincture taken in hot water can be a rapid way to clear any headaches or other acute symptoms of detoxification.	NB: *Do not use at all if you have any metal pins securing fractures, joint replacements or other sources of metal within the body. Only for use once all metal is removed from the mouth.* Because Cilantro mobilizes toxins out of storage it must only be taken in concert with Chlorella to avoid retoxification and you should have been taking Chlorella for at least 2 weeks prior to starting the Cilantro tincture. Do not take around the time of dental procedures as Cilantro will mobilize additional metals out of storage. Suppressed infections can also become symptomatic using Cilantro and may require Samento tincture to clear these. If you experience symptoms such as muscle weakness, fatigue or brain fog decrease or stop taking the Cilantro temporarily and increase the Chlorella. Keep Cilantro tincture out of the reach of children.

Amalgam Removal

Please see chapter 18 for the recommended supplement protocol and other important information. Once your tissues have been significantly detoxified and your amalgam fillings removed, then you can proceed to the post-amalgam removal detoxification protocol.

Figure 37: Summary of post-amalgam removal detoxification protocol 1

Supplement	Breakfast	Lunch	Evening meal
Multimineral/vitamin	1–2 caps	—	1–2 caps
Vitamin C	1g*	1g*	1g*
Fish oils/flax seed oil	2–3 caps	2–3 caps	2–3 caps
Digestive enzymes	(1–2 tabs)	1–2 tabs	1–2 tabs
Psyllium husks	1 tsp	—	1 tsp
Selenium	1 cap	—	1 cap
Vitamin E	1 cap	1 cap	1 cap
Milk thistle	1 cap	1 cap	1 cap
Chlorella pyrenoidosa	3 tabs	3 tabs	3 tabs
Samento tincture	10 drops	(10 drops)†	10 drops
Alpha lipoic acid	1 cap	—	—
Cilantro tincture	5–10 drops‡	5–10 drops‡	5–10 drops‡

* Best taken away from Chlorella
† Introduce third dose after 6 months
‡ See cautions increase slowly from 5 to 10 drops per dose

Post-Amalgam Removal

Three different post-amalgam removal protocols are offered. The first is an extension of the pre-amalgam removal detoxification protocol and is detailed in figure 36 and summarized in figure 37. The second uses Heavy Metal Detox (HMD) and is outlined in figure 38 and summarized in figure 39. The third and last uses the chemical chelator Meso-2, 3-Dimercaptosuccinic acid (DMSA) and is detailed in figure 40 and summarized in figure 41. Chelation (pronounced key-lay-shun) refers to the use of a synthetic substance (a chelator) that can enclose heavy metals within its ring-like structure, thus enabling excretion. You may wish to use all of the suggested protocols at different times for a period of weeks or months, because no one supplement or approach will work in all body compartments and on all forms of mercury. All these protocols involve mobilizing mercury out of the less accessible body compartments, including the cell organelles, the fatty tissue and the brain. It is important that the organs of excretion are supported during this phase to prevent retoxification. You may need to follow these protocols for one to two years until you actually feel fully well. It is this phase of treatment that should see a noticeable improvement in physical, mental and psychological well-being. Some feel that it is best to exhaust the natural options offered in protocols 1 and 2 before using synthetic chemicals to remove mercury. Also, both protocols 2 and 3 employ urinary excretion of mercury and are best avoided if there are any pre-existing bladder or kidney problems.

Figure 38 : Post-amalgam removal detoxification protocol 2

Supplement	Benefits	Cautions
Multimineral/vitamin Dose: Follow manufacturer's recommendations.	See figure 27	See figure 27
Vitamin C Dose: 1g three times a day.	See figure 27	See figure 27
Fish oils/flax seed oil Dose: 500mg three times a day.	See figure 27	See figure 27
Digestive enzymes Dose: 1–2 tabs with meals.	See figure 27	See figure 27
Psyllium husks Dose: 1 tsp twice a day.	See figure 29	See figure 29
Selenium Dose: 1 cap once a day.	See figure 29	See figure 29
Vitamin E Dose: 1 cap three times a day.	See figure 29	See figure 29
Chlorella pyrenoidosa Dose: 3 x 500mg tabs three times a day.	See figure 29	See figure 29
Samento tincture Dose: 10 drops three times a day (increase from twice a day).	See figure 29	See figure 29
HMD Organic Lavage Tincture containing milk thistle and dandelion. For more information or to order contact: www.heavymetaldetox.net. Dose: 25 drops three times a day (see cautions).	Aids detoxification via the liver, kidney and lymph.	Introduce *before* the HMD tincture (below) starting with *one quarter* of the recommended dose, increase slowly and then maintain the dose tolerated. If unwelcome detoxification reactions occur reduce HMD tincture dosage first before reducing the Organic Lavage dose.
Heavy Metal Detox (HMD) HMD tincture contains Chlorella vulgaris, Cilantro tincture and Chlorella growth factor. For more information or to order contact: www.heavymetaldetox.net. Dose: 50 drops three times a day before food (see cautions).	Chelates metals from all body compartments, enhances the growth of friendly bacteria and aids immune function.	Start with *a few drops* three times a day and *increase slowly* to tolerance. Drink plenty of water whilst taking this product. See cautions under Cilantro tincture (figure 36). Detoxification reactions may occur.

Figure 39: Summary of post-amalgam removal detoxification protocol 2

Supplement	Breakfast	Lunch	Evening meal
Multimineral/vitamin	1–2 caps	—	1–2 caps
Vitamin C	1g*	1g*	1g*
Fish oil/flax seed oil	2–3 caps	2–3 caps	2–3 caps
Digestive enzymes	1–2 tabs	1–2 tabs	1–2 tabs
Psyllium husks	1 tsp	—	1 tsp
Selenium	1 cap	—	—
Vitamin E	1 cap	1 cap	1 cap
Chlorella pyrenoidosa	3 tabs	3 tabs	3 tabs
Samento tincture	10 drops	10 drops	10 drops
Heavy Metal Detox	50 drops†	50 drops†	50 drops†
HMD Organic Lavage	25 drops	25 drops	25 drops

* Ideally take vitamin C away from Chlorella
† See cautions figure 38

Whilst many of the symptoms of detoxification may be unwelcome (see chapter 19) they are a necessary part of recovery. However, there is absolutely no point in pulling more mercury out of storage than your body can detoxify and this only leads to retoxification (whereby toxins are redeposited) and may make you feel unwell – possibly for months at a time because of the long half-life of mercury in circulation. Particularly with the post-amalgam removal protocols, it is best to start tentatively with a *fraction of the recommended doses* and *work upwards gradually* until you find a level of detoxification that you can sustain over the long term.

If you cannot afford or cannot face having all your amalgam fillings replaced, then follow the pre-amalgam removal detoxification protocol *for at least 8 months* before switching to the post-amalgam removal detoxification protocols. This decreases the mercury in accessible compartments before further mobilizing mercury out of the tissues. In this instance, protocols 2 and 3 are to be preferred as the use of Cilantro tincture may mobilize mercury from the amalgam fillings into the tissues.

Repair and Maintenance

Finally, figure 42 suggests supplements for aiding repair of the gastrointestinal tract once the post-amalgam removal detoxification process is complete and figure 43 suggests a minimum maintenance protocol thereafter.

Figure 40: Post-amalgam removal detoxification protocol 3

Supplement	Benefits	Cautions

3 DAYS: CHELATION PHASE

Meso-2, 3-dimercaptosuccinic acid (DMSA)

Supplement	Benefits	Cautions
This is a synthetic chemical that chelates heavy metals for excretion in the urine and faeces. It is sold by Thorne as Captomer 100 (100mg DMSA). Follow the renewal protocol below between chelations and do not undertake any other detoxification whilst using Captomer. **Dose:** Take 1 Captomer 100 capsule for every 10kg (approx 20lb) of body weight, spaced throughout the day. Cycle the product 3 days on 11 days off. Start with a reduced dose and work upwards. If you are very sick you may wish to start with a small 'test' dose, reduce the chelation phase and increase the renewal period between doses.	Mobilizes toxic metals from all body compartments including the brain.	May require a prescription, and supervision when using this product is highly recommended. You may feel bad or experience brain fog when using this product as metals are mobilized from storage. Plan for days 2 and 3 to be over a quiet weekend until you have completed several cycles. Pain near the navel is a reported side effect.
Vitamin C **Dose:** 2g twice a day	See figure 27	See figure 27
Digestive enzymes **Dose:** 1–2 tabs with meals	See figure 27	See figure 27
Psyllium husks **Dose:** 1 tsp twice a day	See figure 27	See figure 27
Chlorella pyrenoidosa **Dose:** 2 x 500mg tablets 3 times a day	See figure 29	See figure 29
Whey protein formulation **Dose:** As recommended	See figure 32	See figure 32
Milk thistle **Dose:** 1 cap three times a day	See figure 29	See figure 29

Figure 40: cont.

Supplement	Benefits	Cautions
11 DAYS: RENEWAL PHASE		
Multimineral/vitamin Dose: As recommended.	See figure 27	See figure 27
Vitamin C Dose: 2g twice a day.	See figure 27	See figure 27
Fish oils/flax seed oil Dose: 500mg 3 times a day.	See figure 27	See figure 27
Digestive enzymes Dose: 1–2 tablets with meals.	See figure 27	See figure 27
Psyllium husks Dose: 1 tsp twice a day.	See figure 29	See figure 29
Chlorella pyrenoidosa Dose: 6 x 125mg tablets 3 times a day.	See figure 29	See figure 29
Whey protein formulation Dose: As recommended.	See figure 32	See figure 32
Milk thistle Dose: 1 cap 3 times a day.	See figure 29	See figure 29
Thorne's Heavy Metal Support Dose: 2 caps twice a day.	Replaces minerals and nutrients lost during chelation and restores the kidneys.	Do not take whilst chelating.

Vibrational Remedies

The use of vibrational remedies, such as Bach (pronounced 'batch') Flower Remedies, aids the gentle release of the emotions which have trapped metals and toxins within your system and their use is a great adjunct to treatment and is *highly recommended* throughout the *entire course of treatment*. These remedies exert a gentle effect over time (although this may not be immediately obvious to you) and they can also be taken to relieve an acute situation. Either seek the help of someone trained in this area or select the essence most appropriate to your emotional disposition at any given time. For instance, the Bach flower essence Olive aids feelings of exhaustion and Gentian helps with despair. Don't be frightened of these remedies, since we all have a little of all these

Figure 41: Summary of post-amalgam removal detoxification protocol 3

Supplements	3 DAYS: CHELATION PHASE			11 DAYS: RENEWAL PHASE		
	Breakfast	Lunch	Evening meal	Breakfast	Lunch	Evening meal
Multimineral/ vitamin	—	—	—	1–2 tabs	—	1–2 tabs
Vitamin C	2g	—	2g	2g	—	2g
Fish oils/flax seed oil	—	—	—	2–3 caps	2–3 caps	2–3 caps
Digestive enzymes	1–2 tabs	1–2 tabs	1–2 tabs	1–2 tabs	1–2 tabs	1–2 tabs
Psyllium husks	1 tsp	—	1 tsp	1 tsp	—	1 tsp
Chlorella pyrenoidosa	2 tabs	2 tabs	2 tabs	2 tabs	2 tabs	2 tabs
Whey protein formulation	1 scoop	—	1 scoop	1 scoop	—	1 scoop
Milk thistle	1 cap	1 cap	1 cap	1 cap	1 cap	1 cap
Captomer 100	(2 caps)*	(2 caps)*	(2 caps)*	—	—	—
Heavy Metal Support	—	—	—	2 caps	—	2 caps

* See figure 40, DMSA cautions

emotions; you can only benefit from using them. By gently releasing a variety of 'historic' emotions in this way, the toxins originally associated with these traumas are released and can be detoxified. A guide is available at www.thenaturalrecovery plan.com. Stockists will have a printed guide available and possibly a knowledgeable member of staff too. Muscle testing or dowsing can be used to determine the essence required and the dosage (see Appendix). Typical doses are four drops four times daily or you can dispense them into your water bottle to drink during the day. You can also mix these essences, although taking more than six vibrational remedies at any one time is best avoided.

Tinctures

The Bach Flower Remedies and many of the tinctures recommended are provided in an alcohol base. Some FRS sufferers who are very sensitive to even tiny amounts of alcohol can still use these essences and tinctures by dispensing them into hot (but not boiling) water and leaving for a few minutes for the alcohol to evaporate.

Figure 42: Suggested supplements for repair phase

Supplement	Benefits	Cautions
Aloe vera As juice or capsules. Use high content products that have been hand processed and contain no bitters (which can cause diarrhoea). Dose: Follow manufacturer's instructions.	For general cleansing and intestinal healing.	Use before 'use by' date. Test on skin before consuming as some people are allergic to aloe vera.
Whey protein formulation Dose: Follow manufacturer's instructions.	See figure 32	See figure 32
L-Glutamine Dose: Follow manufacturer's instructions.	An amino acid that promotes gastrointestinal repair and maintenance and is a component of glutathione.	Not recommended during pregnancy and breastfeeding.
Deglycyrrhizinated liquorice (DGL) Dose: Follow manufacturer's instructions.	DGL promotes gastrointestinal healing and blood supply and is protective of the mucosa.	See cautions on product.
Metagenics' Ultraclear Sustain Powdered mix providing a total nutrient blend for gastrointestinal support. Dose: Follow manufacturer's instructions.	Provides the fats and amino acids required to support mucosal health and FOS to promote healthy flora.	Ensure that this product when taken in combination with other products does not exceed the RDA of vitamin A.
N-acetyl glucosamine (NAG) Dose: Follow manufacturer's instructions.	Aids intestinal healing and promotes musculoskeletal health.	See cautions on product.
Probiotics Dose: Follow manufacturer's instructions.	Aids healthy intestinal flora.	See cautions on product. Refrigerate and use before specified date.

Figure 43: Suggested maintenance protocol

Supplements	Breakfast	Lunch	Evening meal
SUGGESTED			
Multimineral/vitamin	1–2 caps	—	—
Vitamin C	1g	—	1g
Fish oils/flax seed oils	2–3 caps	—	—
Chlorella pyrenoidosa	1 tabs	—	1 tabs
OPTIONAL			
Digestive enzymes	—	1 tab	1 tab
Probiotics	1–2 caps	—	1–2 caps
Psyllium husks	1 tsp	—	—

Chapter 18

Dental Work

In order to completely recover your health and to go on to live into a vigorous old age, you may need to commit to having some dental work done (depending upon your current status). This aspect of treatment should not be undertaken lightly because:

- There are often significant costs involved.
- There is often quite a lot of trauma and discomfort involved in possibly having work that has been placed over a lifetime replaced wholesale, especially whilst you may be relatively unwell.
- You may need to travel some distance to see a dentist skilled and knowledgeable in this area.
- This work may also require a considerable commitment in terms of time, not only for yourself but for anyone who may need to accompany you.
- There may be additional expenses such as fees for laboratory testing, intravenous chelating agents or anaesthetist's charges.
- You need to be on a systematic detoxification programme before, during and for some considerable time after dental treatment.
- If not managed effectively, your health can deteriorate even further.

Amalgam Replacement

> *Tolle causam.* (Find the cause.)
>
> **The foundational principle of naturopathic medicine**

The first common sense rule of treatment for any illness is to remove the cause of the problem, if possible. However, all studies show that the removal or placing of amalgam fillings increases the amount of mercury in circulation for many months afterwards. For this reason, a lot of dentists will not replace amalgam fillings without good reason and, of course, the current official line is that the mercury in amalgam does not pose a health threat. In any event, the replacement of amalgam fillings should not be attempted until a lot of your toxic metal load has been dealt with and you are substantially well enough. Careful replacement of amalgam fillings can help some people practically overnight, but if performed without due care or at the wrong time, it can also make some sick people a whole lot worse. This is a specialist job and whilst any dentist should have the technical ability to do the work, not all are aware of the serious health implications of what they are doing in someone whose health is already seriously compromised by mercury toxicity. Some specialist dentists will test the galvanic charges on your amalgam fillings and then remove them in sequence – from those with the strongest negative galvanic charge (which are thought to emit the most mercury vapour) to the least reactive. If you can't afford to have all your fillings replaced, you may at least choose to address the worst offenders on this basis. Alternatively, some authorities recommend removing one filling at a time and spacing the appointments *at least six weeks* apart to reduce any single exposure to mercury vapour.

To find a dentist knowledgeable about amalgam replacement, either ask around, contact one of the organizations listed in the Useful Contacts section or try an Internet search. It is worth ringing the dental practice and asking for an information pack. The dentist concerned should have done amalgam removal courses and ideally would be running a dedicated amalgam-free practice. Any dentist who takes this work seriously should be equally serious about protecting themselves and their staff by taking supplements and using protective equipment. However much you may like your regular dentist, if you have decided to have your amalgam fillings replaced, go and see someone who is an expert in this area.

Recommended Technique

- The dentist should use a rubber dam (a rubber sheet that isolates the tooth/teeth being worked on and serves as a barrier).
- The dentist should provide oxygen while removing the filling(s), and use a nose piece or a damp cloth over the nose.
- Some test the galvanic charges on your amalgam fillings and then remove them in sequence.
- The dentist should have prescribed (or have referred you to someone who has prescribed) various supplements for use before, during and for quite a long time after removal of your amalgam fillings.
- It is thought by some that the immune system has a 7-day cycle and that it can overcome an insult on day 1, but if then further assaulted 14, or especially 21 days later, may be unable to recover. For this reason, try to avoid booking regular weekly appointments.

- Some dentists use intravenous chelating agents during amalgam removal such as 2,3-dimercapto-1-propane sulphonate (DMPS), dimercaptosuccinic acid (DMSA), ethylenediaminetetraacetic acid (EDTA) and/or vitamin C.
- The dentist may use an adrenaline-free local anaesthetic or Carbocaine, which contains only water and anaesthetic, because some FRS sufferers can react badly to regular local anaesthetics.
- Ideally, any replacement restorative materials and anaesthetics should be tested before use. This can be done by muscle testing samples, or a laboratory in the USA can conduct a metal-specific memory T-cell test (MSMT) which can determine the immune response to various dental materials.

Alternative Filling Materials

The most common of these is composite, with other more expensive alternatives including various ceramic, glass and cured-composite materials.

Composite

Composite filling material is the material that is most often used as an alternative to amalgam. It is a plastic material with grains of silica (glass) as a filler to give it durability, body and good aesthetics. It is usually placed in small increments and set with a light and then needs to be trimmed and polished.

The Advantages of Composite

Composite has several qualities to recommend it:

- It does not contain mercury, zinc, copper or silver.
- It is not a metal and so is not electrically active.
- Composite is tooth-coloured and so has good aesthetics.
- Composite fillings can be done in one visit directly in the mouth.
- Whilst it is more expensive than amalgam, it is cheaper than alternatives.

The Disadvantages of Composite

However, it is by no means an ideal filling material (because such a material does not exist) and it has problems of its own:

- Composite shrinks on setting and this can lead to leakage of the filling and ultimately to death of the nerve inside the tooth, whereas amalgam corrodes, sealing the gap. This can mean that your teeth are more likely to die and need a root-filling or extraction if you have composite fillings.

- Composite is also not as durable as amalgam. Teeth are not just for show, they are put under a lot of stress and strain over many decades. Composite fillings will most likely need replacing more often and with every replacement the cavity inevitably becomes larger, the tooth becomes weaker and the nerve inside the tooth becomes more and more compromised.
- Another issue is that the composite filling material is a monomer paste (contains short molecules) and the ultraviolet light sets it into a solid polymer (long molecules). The monomer is moderately toxic and it does not all convert to polymer and this can be an irritant to, and also effectively kill, the nerve inside the tooth. Teeth that die in this way can become incredibly painful and hard to anaesthetize.
- Sometimes, just the action of removing and replacing the filling is enough to push a (possibly not terribly healthy) tooth over the edge into requiring either a root canal filling or extraction.
- Composite can wear over time with consequent movement of opposing or adjacent teeth.
- If the filling is large, or cusps (corners) of the tooth are missing then it is not advisable to have a composite filling. This is because it may be necessary to place pins in the remaining tooth to support the filling (which crazes the tooth with cracks and may lead to the nerve dying) and these fillings tend not to survive very well.
- Bits can and do break off composite fillings, but these can usually be patched because composite can be bonded to itself (within reason).
- There is some question over the safety of composite (and some lining materials) because the plastic component may mimic oestrogen. Similar plastic pollutants are thought to be causing feminization of alligators in Florida, for instance. Many composites now contain aluminium so ensure that the composite to be used has been tested or is aluminium-free. Also, the owner will swallow the small glass particles as the filling wears and it is not known if this is safe.
- It is also technically more demanding to place a composite filling. It has to be placed in increments, ideally under a rubber dam, then trimmed and finished – which all means that they cost quite a lot more than an amalgam filling. It can also be difficult to contour the fillings between teeth and get a good contact which will prevent food from packing between adjacent teeth.

Laboratory-Made Composite Restorations

If your dentist suggests it (and finances permitting), tooth-coloured fillings can be made in a laboratory in much the same way as crowns or caps are and then cemented into place in the mouth. This is advisable for the larger fillings and especially if the tooth concerned is either a premolar or molar tooth that has been root-filled and/or has cusps (corners) missing. One material that can be used is a heat-and-light-cured version of the composite that is used in the mouth. This is more wear-resistant, is fully polymerized and cement seals any gap so that leakage is not an issue. Other options include using either a castable glass or a ceramic material. The finish achieved with these techniques will also be aesthetically pleasing, but these materials can fracture in thin section. Some ceramics also have radioactive elements added in order to simulate the fluorescence of natural teeth. Ceramics, in particular, tend to be harder than natural tooth and can lead to wear of the opposing tooth over time. However, because these techniques involve laboratory bills and extra appointments they usually work out to be many times the cost of composite, although they might save you replacement and root-filling costs in the long run. There are now also non-metal alternatives available for metal posts and 'core' materials (used to build up the tooth under a crown).

Some specialist anti-amalgam dentists may have an expensive piece of computerized kit that can scan the prepared tooth in your mouth and then machine a ceramic or glass restoration to fit while you wait. This means that the work can be completed at the same appointment and may work out somewhat cheaper than a laboratory-fabricated ceramic filling. It also saves having to have two lots of anaesthetic and temporary fillings.

Protocol for replacement of Amalgam Fillings

A protocol is suggested in figure 44 but you should follow the advice of your specialist holistic dentist or anyone they may have referred you to.

In particular, make sure that you are not constipated before, during or after amalgam removal, both by eating a fibrous diet and by supplementing with additional fibre such as psyllium husks. Also remember to follow the protocol for *all* the appointments at which you are having amalgam fillings replaced. If treatment involves extractions or any kind of surgery, the supplement Arnica when taken before, during and after treatment aids healing. Using Dr Bach's Rescue Remedy on the day of, and for a few days after treatment, also diminishes the impact of the trauma on the body. If you are under ongoing treatment with a kinesiologist or naturopath, arrange to see them within one week of amalgam removal. Be aware that some people may have a delayed reaction months after their amalgam replacement for reasons explored earlier.

Figure 44: Supplement protocol for amalgam removal

Supplement	Time	Weeks prior	5 days before
Multimineral/vitamin	am	1–2 caps	1–2 caps
	pm	1–2 caps	1–2 caps
Vitamin C tabs/drink	am	1g	1g
	Lunch/after	1g	1g
	pm	1g	1g
Fish oils/flax seed oil	am	2–3 caps	2–3 caps
	Lunch/after	2–3 caps	2–3 caps
	pm	2–3 caps	2–3 caps
Digestive enzymes	am	1–2 tabs	1–2 tabs
	Lunch/after	1–2 tabs	1–2 tabs
	pm	1–2 tabs	1–2 tabs
Psyllium husks	am	1 tsp	1 tsp
	Lunch/after	–	1 tsp
	pm	1 tsp	1 tsp
Selenium	am	1 cap	1 cap
	Lunch/after	–	1 cap
	pm	1 cap	1 cap
Vitamin E	am	1 cap	1 cap
	Lunch/after	1 cap	1 cap
	pm	1 cap	1 cap
Milk thistle	am	1 cap	2 caps
	Lunch/after	1 cap	–
	pm	1 cap	2 caps
Chlorella pyrenoidosa	am	3 tabs	3 tabs
	Lunch/after	3 tabs	3 tabs
	pm	3 tabs	3 tabs
Samento tincture*	am	10 drops	–
	pm	10 drops	–
NAC†	Before	–	–
	During	–	–
	Lunch/after	–	–
	pm	–	–
Ionic selenium‡	Before/am	–	–
	During/lunch	–	–
	After/pm	–	–
Activated charcoal capsules	am	–	–
	pm	–	–
Milk or soy milk	am	–	–
	pm	–	–

* Optional

† If taking NAC discontinue 5 days before (may interfere with anaesthetic)

‡ Rinsing with ionic selenium (diluted one part to five parts water) helps to prevent the passage of mercury vapour into the brain.

Figure 44: cont.

2 days before	Day of removal	For 2 days after	For 5 days after	After 5 days
1–2 caps	1–2 caps	1–2 caps	1–2 caps	1–2 caps
1–2 caps	1–2 caps	1–2 caps	1–2 caps	1–2 caps
–	–	2g	1g	1g
–	4g	2g	1g	1g
–	2g	2g	1g	1g
2–3 caps	2–3 caps	2–3 caps	2–3 caps	2–3 caps
2–3 caps	2–3 caps	2–3 caps	2–3 caps	2–3 caps
2–3 caps	2–3 caps	2–3 caps	2–3 caps	2–3 caps
1–2 tabs	1–2 tabs	1–2 tabs	1–2 tabs	1–2 tabs
1–2 tabs	1–2 tabs	1–2 tabs	1–2 tabs	1–2 tabs
1–2 tabs	1–2 tabs	1–2 tabs	1–2 tabs	1–2 tabs
1 tsp	1 tsp	1 tsp	1 tsp	1 tsp
1 tsp	1 tsp	1 tsp	1 tsp	–
1 tsp	1 tsp	1 tsp	1 tsp	1 tsp
1 cap	1 cap	1 cap	1 cap	1 cap
1 cap	1 cap	1 cap	1 cap	–
1 cap	1 cap	1 cap	1 cap	1 cap
1 cap	2 caps	1 cap	1 cap	1 cap
1 cap	–	1 cap	1 cap	–
1 cap	2 caps	1 cap	1 cap	1 cap
2 caps	2 caps	2 caps	2 caps	1 cap
–	–	–	–	1 cap
2 caps	2 caps	2 caps	2 caps	1 cap
4 tabs	4 tabs	4 tabs	4 tabs	3 tabs
4 tabs	4 tabs	4 tabs	4 tabs	3 tabs
4 tabs	4 tabs	4 tabs	4 tabs	3 tabs
–	–	–	–	10 drops
–	–	–	–	10 drops
–	–	2 caps	2 caps	–
–	–	–	–	–
–	2 caps	2 caps	2 caps	–
–	2 caps	2 caps	2 caps	–
–	Rinse	Rinse	–	–
–	Rinse	Rinse	–	–
–	Rinse	Rinse	–	–
1 cap	3 caps	–	–	–
1 cap	3 caps	–	–	–
–	1–2 glasses	–	–	–
–	–	–	–	–

Beyond Amalgam Removal

Metals

It depends how sick you are and how much money you can throw at the problem, but some holistic dentists recommend *removal of all metals* and replacement with alternatives to eliminate galvanic currents (chapter 9), metal toxicity and interference with meridian energy flows. This means replacing not only amalgam fillings, but also all crowns, bridges, implants, posts, pins and any dentures incorporating metals.

Root-Fillings

Some authorities also suggest removal of all root-filled teeth. Again, it depends how sick you are, but it might be worth considering. A kinesiologist or a practitioner using some form of biofeedback such as the Vega machine might be able to give you an indication of whether a root-filled tooth is a likely causative factor or not before you take the irreversible step of extraction (also refer to figure 6). Certainly any teeth you know to be a problem such as those with an occasional infection, draining sinus (a little channel through the bone which will appear like an oozing pimple) or with compromised bone support should be extracted. Additionally, any teeth that appear on x-ray to have poor root-fillings should either be re-root-filled or considered for extraction. Dr Weston Price (see chapter 8) found that kidney and heart disease were the disorders that were most responsive to removal of root-filled teeth. More recent evidence also particularly implicates root-filled teeth as a causative factor in diabetes. Dentists who have specialized training in root-fillings are known as endodontists and you may need to request a referral for this treatment. If you have ever had a retrograde amalgam root-filling (a surgical treatment sealing the root canal from the root tip) you will need to decide whether repeating minor surgery to keep a compromised tooth is worth it in light of your general health.

Cavitations

Neuralgia-inducing cavitational osteonecrotic (NICO) lesions or cavitations are cavities within the jawbone that have been left by extracted teeth, most often wisdom teeth. If x-rays indicate that this might be an issue for you, find a specialist dentist who can perform the minor surgery of opening up and cleaning out the affected area. Some dentists with a special interest in this area may also have a piece of equipment known as a Cavitat. This provides an ultrasonographic print-out of the quality of the bone surrounding the teeth and indicates the presence of necrotic lesions or cavitations with a high degree of accuracy. A kinesiologist or muscle testing (see Appendix) may also be able to establish whether this is a causative factor in your FRS.

Joining the Dots

The US anti-amalgam dentist, Dr Hal Huggins, refers to doing all of the above as total dental revision (TDR) and claims to get good results for some very sick people. It might be worth trying to do some detective work and write down when you had dental work done (to the best of your recollection) and when your FRS symptoms appeared. See if there is any obvious culprit such as a recent root-filling, placement of a crown or bridge, or removal of a wisdom tooth that might have been associated with the onset of symptoms. Metal framework crowns and bridges (which may be covered in porcelain) placed over amalgam 'cores' may be particular suspects and your dental records will reveal whether this applies to you. Also consider that work done on a tooth that has subsequently been extracted may have initiated the causative processes of FRS. The development of white bands or Mees' lines on the finger- or toenails and raised cholesterol levels may also occur in response to recent exposure to heavy metals and these may also act as clues to help point you in the right direction. Hal Huggins claims that the vast majority of his patients report relief of allergies, bloating, migraine, digestive and urinary tract problems and fatigue with removal of their amalgam fillings according to his protocols.

Chapter 19
The Healing Journey

If you're going through hell, keep going.

Sir Winston Churchill

The healing journey is a bit like a maze that you have got lost in over the years, and to return to health your body needs to retrace its footsteps. This means that the body releases both the toxins and associated emotions in reverse order in 'layers' as you unravel the mess. Whilst this process is enabled by releasing emotional issues and supporting the processes of detoxification using supplements, it is ultimately governed by the incredible intelligence of the body. The particular manifestations are usually hard to predict because neither practitioner nor client are aware of what toxins have compromised which systems and when. Recovery requires that you *deliberately retoxify* your body by pulling potent toxins out of 'safe' storage in various body compartments in order to detoxify and excrete them. On a good day this may mean that you feel just a little below par, but if you are really detoxifying significant quantities of toxins there are likely to be some unpleasant side effects. The speed with which you can detoxify depends upon how compromised your organs of detoxification and excretion are, and to attempt to accelerate the process without professional help can result in serious damage to these organs. Do not for one minute underestimate how noxious these incredibly toxic substances are and the harm that they can do to a biological system.

One of the naturopathic principles is that strong systems react strongly and weak systems react weakly. This means that as your body gains strength it is able to pull more toxins out of storage for processing. This often feels as though you are taking one step forward and two steps back. However, be assured that if you are doing all the right things, you are making progress. Because mercury has a half-life in the circulation of 70 days this means that even when supplementing it takes about eight months to process 90 per cent of any initial amount of circulating mercury. Many become discouraged and give up somewhere on their healing journey, but the prize goes to those who, like the tortoise, just keep on going. A lot of the time it may feel as though nothing much is happening – and the remainder of the time you may wish that nothing were!

Symptoms of Detoxification

> What is impossible to see from the viewpoint of those who believe in cures is that the very symptoms the good doctors have suppressed and turned into chronic disease were the body's only means of correcting the problem! The so-called 'disease' was the only 'cure' possible!

Dr Philip Chapman

The symptoms of detoxification associated with the four routes of excretion (five in menstruating women) are listed in figure 45. These are all signs that treatment is working, although the particular symptoms may not be very welcome. Rashes often occur at the beginning and end points of the energy meridians, often, but not exclusively, on the face, hands and feet. In order to be able to interpret your detoxification

Figure 45: Routes of detoxification

Detoxification route	Symptom
Faeces	Change in bowel habits; stools become loose; diarrhoea; different colour; flatulence.
Urine	Dark and/or pungent odour; burning on urination.
Breath	Bad breath as gases are detoxified from lungs. NB: If your breath smells consistently bad, then you may want to investigate the possibility that you have gum disease, tooth decay, infected sinuses and/or tonsils or post-nasal drip (where mucous accumulates at the root of the tongue in the throat). Bad breath may also originate from a toxic bowel.
WOMEN ONLY	
Menstrual bleed	Disruption to cycle; nature of bleed may change; blood may become dark and/or clotted.
PERIPHERY	
Skin	In females thrush or other vaginal irritation and in males 'jock' itch. Yeast infections in body creases; athlete's foot as your body expels Candida and other yeasts. You may develop sore and very itchy rashes as toxins are released through the skin. The skin around the eyes typically becomes swollen, itchy and 'cracked' unlike elsewhere on the body. Your outer ear canal may swell and become tender.
Mucosa	Your gums may become tender or swollen – typically in only one section of your mouth. You may develop sores in your nose or ulcers in your mouth. Excessive mucous production may induce a cough. Your tonsils may become swollen and/or sore.
Nails	Your finger- and/or toenails may change colour, developing white patches or lines as toxic metals are released from storage. They may also become either deeply horizontally or vertically ridged and if you have never had half moons these may start to form.

symptoms, figure 46 shows the locations of the meridian end points and some relevant acupuncture points on the extremities and the systems or organs with which they are associated. The organ systems are all related to specific muscles and although this is beyond the scope of this book, this possibility is worth considering if you suddenly experience unexplained muscle weakness, pain or tension. The muscles relating to the gall bladder, for instance, control the knee; those of the endocrine system, the ankle and lower leg; and the kidney, the hip. These are signs that one or more organs systems are in distress and you may need to consult your practitioner or reduce your detoxification if these signs occur. Symptoms such as sharp or recurring pains also typically occur along overactive meridians and figure 47 gives a brief overview of the routes of the meridians. More detailed information is freely available online or in any Traditional Chinese Medicine (TCM) textbook. According to TCM, each organ system comes to the fore at a particular time of the day and these times are shown in figure 48. This accounts for the fluctuating symptoms of FRS, for symptoms that are worse at particular times of the day and can also indicate which organ system is detoxifying. For example, a rash which becomes very itchy in the evening may indicate clearance from the endocrine system or sex organs and sweating between 1 and 3am indicates clearance from, or by, the liver. Touch for Health courses are widely available and are intended as introductory courses in energy management based upon the principles of TCM for laypeople if you would like to learn more about this subject. Regular acupuncture treatments may also help to open the channels of excretion during your detoxification. Finally, Tui Na and Shiatsu massage also works using touch along the meridians to promote and maintain energy flows. If you aren't totally convinced about the existence of these subtle flows, you almost certainly will be after one of these treatments!

Healing Crises

Almost everyone will undergo one or more 'healing crisis' on their journey to health and some of these symptoms can be quite alarming. Amongst many other symptoms, I went deaf for three weeks, was unable to balance or stand for a day and my fingers were either *insanely* itchy, swollen or terribly sore with the loss of various fingernails and sloughing skin for *many, many* months. Hold firm when these things happen, because happen they will and there really is no other lasting solution that will see you recover your health other than to pass through them. It is always going to be a compromise between severe detoxification symptoms experienced over a short period of time and less severe symptoms experienced over a longer period of time. It's your choice, but if you want to get better as quickly as possible, then you may necessarily

Figure 46: Meridian end points and related acupuncture points

Location	Associated meridian
Face	
Inner eyelid	Bladder
Beneath the eye	Stomach
Outer eyebrow	Endocrine system/thyroid
Outer corner of the eye	Gall bladder
In front of the ear	Small intestine
Where cheek meets nose	Large intestine
Hands	
Back of thumb	Lungs
Back of first finger	Large intestine
Palm side second finger	Sex organs
Back of third finger	Endocrine system/thyroid
Back of little finger	Small intestine
Palm side of little finger	Heart
Feet	
Upper big toe	Spleen (pancreas)
Between first and second toes	Liver
Fourth toe	Gall bladder
Little toe	Bladder
Ball of foot	Kidney

Location	Acupuncture points
Hands	
Outside little finger	Left leg
Inside little finger	Right leg
Little finger aspect of ring finger	Left arm/shoulder
Middle finger aspect ring finger	Right arm/shoulder

have some rapid detoxifying to do. On the plus side, these reactions are proof positive that what you are doing is proving effective and that your body is strong enough to do the work. Rashes on your fingers, for instance, may indicate that toxins have travelled from deep storage to be released at your extremities. Excretion through the skin is the best way the body can guarantee elimination of toxins since discharge into both the bile and urine allow for possible reuptake. Having regular colonics throughout treatment will also help to prevent the reabsorption of toxins by the extensive nerve plexus of the alimentary tract and the circulation and aid elimination. Your body is prioritizing detoxification of the *100 trillion cells* of which it is composed and this process has to be respected. So, if at all possible just permit this final release rather than frustrating the body's attempts to rid itself of its toxic burden. In my experience, with every wave of nasty detoxification symptoms you will access a proportionately higher level of vitality – although that may not be obvious to you at the time. If you are experiencing particularly troublesome symptoms please refer to figure 49 and review the various

Figure 47: The routes of the meridians

Meridian	Begins	Route	Ends
FRONT OF BODY			
Central (brain) [reservoir]	Pubis	Midline of body	Under lower lip
Kidney	Ball of foot	Inside ankle–inside calf–inside thigh –just lateral to midline of body	Clavicle lateral to midline
Liver	Between first and second toes	Between inside and front of calf and thigh –lateral to pubis–mid lateral torso	Mid flat part of ribs under breast
Spleen (immune/ pancreas)	Top big toe	Runs up inner foot–inside midline lower leg and knee–runs up mid thigh–mid hip –lateral torso	Side of body between armpit and waist
Stomach	Under eye	Loops over cheek and eye–side nose–mid neck–turns laterally to nipple–either side of midline torso–lateral to middle of front of leg	Top second toe
ARMS			
Heart	Armpit	Runs along underside of arm	Palm side little finger
Circulation sex (sex hormones)	Nipple	Inside of arm–mid palm	Palm side of second finger
Lung	Above and lateral to nipple	Front of arm–inside wrist	Palm side of thumb
Large intestine	Back first finger	Back arm–side neck	Side nostril
Triple warmer (thyroid)	Back third finger	Back/inside arm–side neck–over ear	Outside eyebrow
Small intestine	Outer edge of little finger	Outside wrist–elbow–back arm–shoulder –side/back neck–cheek	In front of ear
SIDE BODY			
Gall bladder	Lateral to eye	Complex route over temple/side of head/ behind ear–back neck–over shoulder –side body–side leg–outside ankle	Top of fourth toe
BACK BODY			
Bladder	Inner eye	Up over top of head–back neck–takes two routes over torso: one either side of spine/coccyx and one over shoulder/lateral to spine and mid buttock–mid back leg –outer border of foot	Top little toe
Governing [reservoir]	Anus	Spine–over top of head–midline of face	Above upper lip

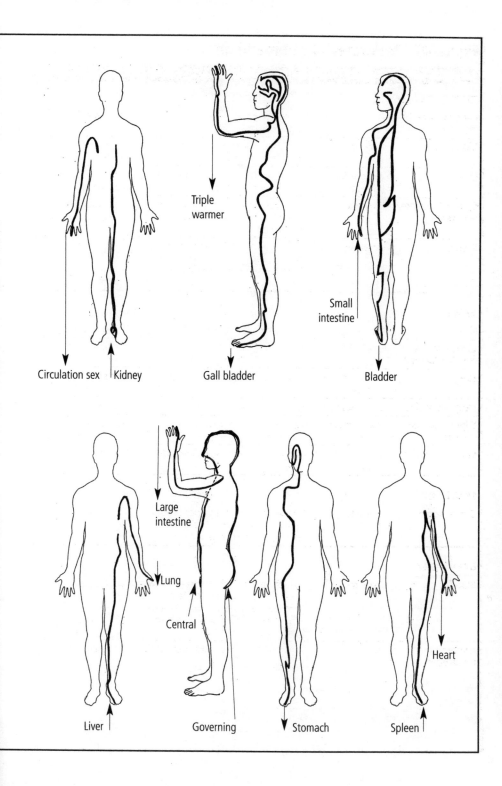

Circulation sex | Kidney

Triple warmer

Gall bladder

Small intestine

Bladder

Large intestine

Lung

Central

Liver

Governing

Stomach

Spleen

Heart

Figure 48: Peak activity of organ systems

MORNING		AFTERNOON	
Time	Organ system	Time	Organ system
1–3am	Liver	1–3pm	Small intestine
3–5am	Lung	3–5pm	Bladder
5–7am	Large intestine	5–7pm	Kidney
7–9am	Stomach	7–9pm	Sex hormones
9–11am	Spleen	9–11pm	Endocrine (thyroid)
11am–1pm	Heart	11pm–1am	Gall bladder

Figure 49: Troubleshooting healing crises

Problem	Solution
Are you drinking enough water?	Ensure that you are drinking at least two litres of water a day and increase this if you want to assist your body to flush through toxins.
Have you drunk a different type or amount of alcohol to usual?	Cut out all alcohol, reduce amount or change type of alcohol consumed.
Are you constipated?	Ensure that you are eating a fibrous diet and if you are not already supplementing with an additional source of fibre, consider doing so. Consider whether you could have eaten a food to which you are intolerant, e.g. dairy. Have a colonic or use Epsom salts.
Have you introduced any foods recently?	Think about it and eliminate the food and try re-introducing it at a later date.
Have you started taking any pharmaceuticals or supplements and/or changed doses recently?	A reaction could either be because a particular substance does not agree with you or because it is promoting a detoxification reaction. Ensure that you are taking enough Chlorella to bind the toxins being excreted and if necessary *increase* the amount you are taking. Other than Chlorella, consider the possibilities and either reduce the amount, replace with a similar product or remove any recently introduced substances.
Are you eating enough protein?	Ensure that you are eating at least two and ideally three portions of high-quality animal protein a day.
Have you relaxed with regard to buying and cooking nutritious foods?	Reinstitute the basics.
Did you feel better just prior to feeling a whole lot worse?	In this instance, the fact that you had become stronger may have enabled your body to tackle another 'layer' of toxins.
Can you remember having this symptom before?	For instance, a sore throat may indicate that you have cleared emotional issues and associated toxins back to the age of five years old when you had tonsillitis.
Can you remember experiencing these emotions before?	You re-experience the shadow of the original emotion so that feeling angry or sad for seemingly no reason may relate back to a time in your life when you felt this way and may give you an indication of what you are clearing.
Are you getting enough rest and sleep?	Treat yourself kindly and make sure that you are getting enough rest, sleep and exercise during this time. Have a bath and go to bed early.

Figure 49: cont.

Problem	Solution
Are you getting enough exercise?	Either increase or reinstate a regular gentle exercise regime.
Are you taking a supplement to aid your organs of detoxification?	You may want to assist your liver and/or kidney function by supplementing a product such as milk thistle and/or dandelion/Uva ursi herbal blends respectively – or to increase your dose if you already taking these supplements.
Are you taking Samento tincture?	If you are experiencing unwelcome detoxification reactions, then it might be a good idea to temporarily reduce or stop your dose of Samento tincture.
Do you feel horrible, but think that it is a detoxification reaction?	Detoxifying baths, saunas, lymphatic drainage, massage and skin brushing may help. Use a chi machine if you have one. Have a colonic. Some authorities recommend excluding all sulphur supplements and foods to prevent retoxification.
Have you developed some new symptom such as tinnitus, headache, neuralgia or muscle aches?	Toxins are being redeposited rather than excreted and you may need to review your supplementation increasing your Chlorella or adding in, or increasing supplements to aid your organs of detoxification such as milk thistle for the liver or dandelion/Uva ursi for the bladder. Discontinue any sulphur supplements such as NAC or MSM. Alternatively or additionally a colonic might help at these times.
Has your urine developed a pink or purple tinge?	A sign of excess porphyrins in the urine – an early sign of the porphyria depicted in the film *The Madness of King George*. Can be associated with digestive/ psychological/nervous disturbances. Drink lots of water, suspend all supplements except for Chlorella and seek the advice of your health professional.

contributory factors. Some contend that the whole of recovery is one long healing crisis and I couldn't really give them an argument!

Different detoxifying agents have different affinities for the toxic metals in their various forms, known as valences. They are also fickle, because having pulled one toxin out of storage they might find a more attractive partner *en route* and dump the original toxic metal which will have to be re-stored. This I think accounts for a lot of the shifting symptoms of both FRS and detoxification as there is a constant flux of toxins being shuffled around the body according to such factors as the time of day and nutrients available.

Psychological Aspects of Recovery

> Hold the ideal of yourself as you long to be, always, everywhere – your ideal of what you long to attain – the ideal of health, efficiency, success.

Orison Swett Marden

Whilst physical detoxification is extremely trying, the emotions experienced whilst detoxifying are horribly confusing. You never know whether you are releasing some ancient emotion or experiencing it in present time. You may come to understand that your emotional body is every bit as real as your physical body – although intangible – and many of the feelings that need to be released are shadows from your past. The good news is that you are finally ready to release them along with the toxins they have 'trapped' in your body. You also need to be prepared for the psychiatric symptoms such as anxiety, depression, agitation, paranoia, confusion and possibly even feeling suicidal. Understand that these are *symptoms of mercury in circulation and that they will pass.* You may also not be able to make your brain work at all some days and may become clumsy or accident-prone. Some days or weeks may pass in a dream-like blur as mercury affects the very nature of consciousness. Understand that it is going to be a long-drawn-out, confusing rollercoaster ride of various symptoms and emotions, and there will be plenty of frustration and impatience and believing it all to be hopeless and a lost cause along the way. There are times when I thought it would *never* end, but equally knew there were no viable options other than to keep going. When the dawn eventually came, it came surprisingly suddenly and unexpectedly, so you literally never know when you are on the verge of a breakthrough.

Try to hold fast to a future vision of yourself – fully recovered and doing something that is meaningful to you, or just enjoying life – during your healing journey. Make it real by pasting your photo onto a picture from a magazine if necessary and either look at it or call it to mind every time you feel discouraged and remind yourself that it is a prize worth attaining. Frankly, nothing in life worth having comes easily and regaining your health – or in my case experiencing health for the first time – after the living nightmare of FRS is particularly sweet. The physical symptoms will clear before the emotional and mental symptoms, with introversion being the last symptom to go. If your body has sustained extensive 'autoimmune' damage, then a full recovery may not prove possible or may require the help of a skilled naturopathic practitioner, but you will still be able to improve your health substantially and prevent further deterioration.

... And Finally

Although there are unpredictable risks inherent in detoxifying these risks can, by and large, be managed – whereas the risks inherent in staying sick are all too predictable. I wish I could tell you that there was an easier way to recover than having to pass through the flames of the fire. However, you and me both, and tens of millions of other FRS sufferers and many billions of others with degenerative and chronic illnesses, have all been victims of the most extensive case of poisoning in the history of the world – ironically perpetrated in the name of health care. I now realize that mercury toxicity took many relatives before their time, my mother's sanity, my father's health and dignity, my fertility and nearly my life … and I am by no means an unusual case. The authorities will eventually have to concede the toxicity of the use of mercury in dental amalgam and vaccinations. The question is how many millions more must suffer terribly before they do? My prayer is that we learn the lessons of FRS as soon as possible and prevent further poisoning of future generations. We can then start to clear up the tremendous damage that has been inflicted upon individuals and the Earth and learn to treat both human physiology and the planetary ecosystem with the respect that they deserve. Finally, you cannot abdicate this responsibility to those you perceive to be powerful. We have to – in the words of Mother Teresa – 'Do it alone, person to person.'

We are the ones we have been waiting for.

Hopi proverb

Appendix

The techniques described below are accessing something far greater than our limited individual knowledge at any given time. Some believe that they are tapping into the individual subconscious, some that they are accessing a higher aspect of the self and some that they are connecting with the collective 'field' of universal consciousness. To those with a left-brain orientation, using these techniques may initially require a leap of faith; however, experience has shown that these answers are reliable when testing is properly conducted. Please suspend your rational 'ego' brain which needs to understand how everything works and try the techniques described below for a practical and usually incontrovertible and revelatory personal demonstration!

If you wish to explore this topic further or receive formal instruction in these techniques, courses in both dowsing and Touch for Health (which offer an introduction to muscle testing and energy management) may be available locally. Alternatively there are DVDs, books and various online videos demonstrating the techniques involved. For further information you may also want to read *Power vs Force* by Dr David Hawkins or *Energy Medicine* by Donna Eden.

Muscle Testing
Two-Person Testing

Two people are required in order to perform this muscle test and the tester should not unduly stress the subject by standing too close to, or looking directly at, the subject while testing. Make sure that there are no distractions (other people, music, pets, etc.) and the subject (and possibly the tester) should remove their glasses, any watches and/or jewellery and any other magnets or crystals. Belt buckles and body piercings – especially metal rings in belly button piercings – may also need to be removed. Both parties should try to be blank slates by putting aside any scepticism, avoiding anticipating any particular response(s) and also not allowing their mind(s) to wander to worries or concerns which may affect the outcome. In fact, it is sometimes better that the tester does not reveal the food being tested, for example, to the subject to avoid this affecting the result.

The Technique

The subject can sit or stand, holding one arm straight horizontally either in front or to their side. Whilst gently holding the subject's other shoulder the tester applies *gentle and brief two-finger pressure* downwards to the wrist of the arm being tested. Alternatively, the subject can stand or lie down with their arm at their side and with the *back of their hand* against their thigh. The tester can then slip their hand between the subject's wrist and body and apply *gentle pressure* to pull the arm away from the body. These tests are assessing *energy flows* within the body and are *not tests of strength*. The most common mistakes are that testers use too much force and that subjects resist too strongly. The tester is simply trying to establish whether the muscles are locking or unlocking in response to the test statement, food or supplement. The tester should warn the subject that they are about to test by saying 'And hold,' and then applying *gentle, steady* pressure and avoiding jerking the arm. To establish that the subject is currently testable either party can place their fingers or hand over the subject's third eye (between their eyebrows) as the tester muscle tests. This should make the test muscle unlock, i.e. generally weaken the subject's energy system.

Calibrating the Response

Establish which response is which by asking, 'Please show me a "yes",' (muscle test) and, 'Please show me a "no",' (test again) and recording or remembering the result. This may change from time to time and individual to individual, so always start each session by establishing these responses. You can then test the subject whilst they first think about someone they love, which may strengthen their energy flows, making them test 'strong', i.e. the muscle 'locks'. Then have the subject think about someone with whom they have a problematic relationship and this may weaken their energy flows and they may test 'weak', i.e. the muscle 'unlocks'. Alternatively, they can state their name ('My name is …') and this being a true statement the muscle being tested should remain strong or 'lock'. Then have the subject state a false name and this being untrue, the body's energies respond and the muscle being tested should go weak or 'unlock'.

Self-Testing

Some people are able to muscle test themselves successfully and one option is to make an 'O' shape using your first finger and thumb on your *non-dominant hand* and then to attempt to break the 'ring' formed by passing the first finger of the opposite hand between the thumb and finger contact. This is a more discreet method to use for testing foods or supplements in a shop, for instance, by holding them or touching them while testing, although it may not prove as reliable as two-person testing. Another method of self-testing involves facing north and holding a test substance (e.g. a bag of flour or a carton of milk) to your solar plexus and seeing whether your body is drawn forwards (a beneficial substance) or responds by recoiling backwards (a detrimental substance). You can use these techniques to dynamically assess changing responses to foodstuffs over time.

Dowsing

Any weighted object on any kind of cord can be used for dowsing; however, crystal dowsing stones suspended on chains are relatively inexpensive, highly portable and the responses are easy to determine. As with muscle testing, the dowser gives binary responses, i.e. 'yes' or 'no' answers. Hold the chain, leaving about 5cm or so (2 inches) over your first finger and setting it in motion and then ask to be shown a 'yes' and then a 'no' response. This may be an anticlockwise motion for one and a clockwise response for the other or a back and forth or side to side motion. Note the response you receive and give thanks for the response. If you fail to get consistent responses you can state, 'Let this be my "yes",' and move the dowser in a particular manner and then, 'Let this be my "no",' and again move the dowser in a different way. Then check this preset response as above.

General Points About Muscle Testing and Dowsing

If the person who is being tested does not respond appropriately either the tester and/or the subject may be dehydrated, and both parties drinking some water may rectify the situation. Sometimes, either a recent meal or geopathic or electromagnetic stress of one or both individuals may throw off test results. Both the tester and the subject can temporarily reset their systems by thumping their thymus gland (upper sternum) once a second or so while thinking of someone they love and smiling. If you cannot get reliable responses at any given time for whatever reason, it is probably best to try again later.

Testing Foods

Foods being tested can be held next to the solar plexus (upper abdomen) of the subject and a strong muscle test (a 'yes' using dowsing) means the food is supportive of health and a weak muscle test (a 'no' using dowsing) means that the food is having a detrimental effect. Artificial sweeteners, margarine and/or cell phones (switched on) universally make almost everyone weaken and can be used to test responsiveness.

Testing Supplements

Supplements too can be held against the subject's solar plexus and muscle tested or the statement, 'It is in my highest interests to take this supplement at this time,' used if dowsing. If a supplement tests positive then state, 'Doses per day ... one, two, three,' (testing for each response) and then, 'Capsules/drops/tablets per dose ... one, two, three,' testing again. Check the answer by stating, 'Two capsules to be taken three times a day,' (for example) and you may also wish to check for how long by stating, 'To be taken for one week, two weeks,' testing responses. As the body requests the supplements it requires, place them on the subject's lap or near to their body. Obviously, check the manufacturer's instructions with regards to dosing and do not exceed recommended doses.

Testing Statements

All statements should be phrased as declarative positive statements in the present tense (not asking about the future) and should not employ words that are subject to interpretation or judgement. Statements need to be phrased so that you can receive a 'yes' or 'no' answer and a good way of phrasing statements is, 'It is in my highest interests to ...' Sometimes the wording of the statement may be problematic and rephrasing the statement or even just changing one word may change the meaning. It may not be appropriate to ask a specific question at a certain time and this should be cleared first by stating, 'It is appropriate to enquire about this topic at this time.' You also cannot use these techniques in an intrusive way to interfere with others' free will, but only in relation to yourself or with the express permission or at the request of another party. Also, appreciate that the answers you get may make no sense at your present level of understanding or because you are currently missing important information. Often people place their own interpretation upon the results and it can be worth documenting the exact questions and responses and referring to them later, when you may come to understand the answers in a completely different light.

Further Reading

Arem, Ridha, MD, *The Thyroid Solution*, Ballantine Publishing, 2007

Batmanghelidj, F, MD, *Your Body's Many Cries For Water: A revolutionary natural way to prevent illness and restore good health*, Global Health Solutions Inc, 2004

Blaylock, Russell L, *Excitotoxins: The taste that kills.* Health Press, 1996

Braden, Gregg, *The Divine Matrix: Bridging time, space, miracles and belief*, Hay House, 2008

Braden, Gregg, *The Spontaneous Healing of Belief: Shattering the paradigm of false limits*, Hay House, 2008

Bradshaw, John, *Family Secrets: What you don't know can hurt you*, Bantam, 1995

Breiner, Mark A, DDS, *Whole-Body Dentistry*, Quantum Health Press, 1999

Budd, Martin, ND, DO, *Why Am I So Tired? Is your thyroid making you ill?* Thorsons, 2000

Castelli, William, MD and Griffin, Glen C, MD, *Good Fat, Bad Fat: Lower your cholesterol and reduce your odds of a heart attack*, Fisher Books, 2000

Chaitow, Leon, ND, DO, *Candida Albicans*, Thorsons, 2003

Chaitow, Leon, ND, DO, *Fibromyalgia And Muscle Pain: Your self-treatment guide*, Thorsons, 2001

Chopra, Dr Deepak, *SynchroDestiny: Harnessing the infinite power of coincidence to create miracles*, Rider Books, 2003

Clark, Hulda Rugehr, PhD, ND, *The Cure For All Diseases*, New Century Press, 2002

Clayton, Paul, PhD, *Health Defence*, Accelerated Learning System, 2004

Coleman, Dr Vernon, *How To Stop Your Doctor Killing You*, European Medical Journal, revised edition 2003

Craggs-Hinton, Christine, *Living With Fibromyalgia: Overcoming common problems*, Sheldon Press, 2000

Cutler, Andrew Hall, PhD, PE, *Amalgam Illness, Diagnosis And Treatment: What you can do to get better.* Available from the author at: www.noamalgam.com

Dalvi, Dr Salmann, *Adrenal Fatigue: A desk reference*, Authors Online, 2003

Diamond, John, *Life Energy: Using the meridians to unlock the hidden power of your emotions*, Continuum, 1990

Dunne, Lavon J, *Nutrition Almanac*, McGraw-Hill, 2002

Durant-Peatfield, Barry, MB, BS, LRCP, MRCS, *Your Thyroid And How To Keep It Healthy: The great thyroid scandal and how to survive it*, Barons Down, 2006

Eden, Donna, *Energy Medicine*, Tarcher Penguin, 2003

Emoto, Masaru, *The Hidden Messages In Water*, Beyond Words Publishing, 2004

Gallo, Fred, PhD and Vincenzi, Harry, EdD, *Energy Tapping: How to rapidly eliminate anxiety, depression, cravings and more using energy psychology*, New Harbinger Publications, 2000

Gamlin, Linda, *The Allergy Bible*, Quadrille, 2005

Gauquelin, Michel, MD, *How Cosmic And Atmospheric Energies Influence Your Health*, Aurora Press, 1971

Gerber, Richard, MD, *Vibrational Medicine*, Bear and Company, 2001

Gittlemen, Ann Louise, MS, CNS, *Guess What Came To Dinner: Parasites and your health*, Avery Press, 2001

Gordon, Rolf, *Are You Sleeping In A Safe Place?* Dulwich Health Society, 1989

Goswami, Amit, PhD, *The Self-Aware Universe: How consciousness creates the material world*, Tarcher, 1995

Halvorsen, Richard, MD, *The Truth About Vaccines: How We Are Used As Guinea Pigs Without Knowing It*, Gibson Square, 2007

Hanley, Jesse Lynn, MD and Deville, Nancy, *Tired Of Being Tired*, Michael Joseph Publishing, 2002

Hawkins, David, MD, PhD, *Power vs Force: The hidden determinants of human behavior*, Hay House, 2007

Hay, Louise, *You Can Heal Your Life*, Hay House, 2004

Hellinger, Bert, *Love's Hidden Symmetry: What makes love work in relationships*, Zeig, Tucker and Co Ltd, 1999

Hightower, Jane, M, MD, *Diagnosis: Mercury. Money, politics and poison*, Island Press, 2009

Holford, Patrick, *The Holford Low GL Diet: Lose weight and feel great in 30 days*, Atria Publishing, 2005

Huggins, Hal A, DDS, MS, *It's All In Your Head: The link between mercury amalgams and illness*, Avery Press, 1993

Huggins, Hal A, DDS, MS and Levy, Thomas E, MD, JD, *Uninformed Consent: The hidden dangers in dental care*, Hampton Press, 1998

Katie, Byron, *Loving What Is: Four questions that can change your life*, Three Rivers Press, 2002

Kirby, David, *Evidence Of Harm: Mercury in vaccines and the autism epidemic – a medical controversy*, St Martin's Griffin, 2005

Klinghardt, Dietrich, MD, PhD, An informative website at www.klinghardtacademy.com.

Kushi, Michi, *Your Body Never Lies*, Square One Publishers, 2007

Lagro-Janssen T et al., 'Breast cancer and hormone-replacement therapy in the Million Women Study', *Lancet*, pp. 419–27, 9 August 2003

Lipton, Bruce, PhD, *The Biology Of Belief: Unleashing the power of consciousness, matter and miracles*, Mountain of Love Publishing, 2005

MacIntyre, Anne, *ME: Chronic Fatigue Syndrome: A practical guide*, Thorsons Health, 1998

Marber, Ian, *The Food Doctor Diet*, Dorling Kindersley, 2004

McTaggart, Lynn, *The Field*, Element, 2003

McTaggart, Lynn, *What Doctors Don't Tell You*, Thorsons Element, 2005

McTaggart, Lynn (ed.), *What Doctors Don't Tell You: Dental ebook*, www.wddty.com

Mendelsohn, Robert, S, MD, *How To Raise A Healthy Child In Spite Of Your Doctor*, Mass Market Paperback, 1987

Mumby, Dr Keith, *The Allergy Handbook*, Thorsons Publishing, 2004

Murphy, Christine (ed.), *The Vaccination Dilemma*, Lantern Books, 2000

Murray, Michael, ND and Pizzorno, Joseph, ND, *Encyclopaedia Of Natural Medicine*, Little Brown, 2002

Myhill, Sarah, MB, BS, *Diagnosing And Treating Chronic Fatigue Syndrome*, available from the author at www.drmyhill.co.uk

Myss, Caroline, PhD, *Anatomy Of The Spirit*, Bantam Books 1997

Myss, Caroline, PhD, *Sacred Contracts: Awakening your full potential*, Bantam Books, 2002

Myss, Caroline, PhD, *Why People Don't Heal And How They Can*, Bantam Books, 1998

Newman, David, R, *Flushed With Success: The bottom line on colonic irrigation*, Cedar Publishing Ltd, 2002

Nugent, Steve, ND, PhD, *How To Survive On A Toxic Planet*, The Alethia Corporation, 2004

Page, Dr Christine, *Frontiers Of Health: How to heal the whole person*, Random House, 1992

Perrin, Raymond, DO, *The Perrin Technique: How to Beat Chronic Fatigue Syndrome/ME*, Hammersmith Press Ltd, 2007

Pert, Candace, PhD, *Molecules Of Emotion*, Pocket Books, 1999

Price, Weston, DDS, *Nutrition And Physical Degeneration*, Price-Pottenger Nutrition, 2008

Rooman, Lily, *All About Chakras: Knowing and activating the body's energy centres*, Astrolog, 2003

Sahelian, Ray, MD, *DHEA: A practical guide*, Avery Press, 1999

Scaer, Robert, C, *The Body Bears the Burden: Trauma, dissociation, and disease*, The Haworth Press, 2007

Shames, Richard and Shames, Karilee, *Feeling Fat, Fuzzy Or Frazzled?* Hudson Street Press, 2006

Shomon, Mary J, *Living Well With Hypothyroidism*, Quill Publishing, 2005

Shomon, Mary J, *Living Well With Chronic Fatigue Syndrome And Fibromyalgia*, Quill Publishing, 2004

Siegel, Bernie, MD, *Love, Medicine And Miracles*, Harper Perennial, 1999

St Amand, R Paul and Craig Marek, Claudia, *What Your Doctor May Not Tell You About Fibromyalgia: The revolutionary treatment that can reverse the disease*, Little, Brown and Co, 2006

Smith, Dr Tom, *How To Successfully Cope With Thyroid Problems*, Wellhouse Publishing Ltd, 2001

Thie, John, DC, *Touch For Health: A practical guide to natural health with acupressure touch and massage*, DeVorss Publications, 2002

Thurnell-Read, Jane, *Geopathic Stress And Subtle Energy*, Life Work Potential, 2006

Thurnell-Read, Jane, *Geopathic Stress: How earth energies affect our lives*, Element Aurora, 2003

Timbrell, John, *Principles Of Biochemical Toxicology*, fourth edition, Informa Healthcare, 2009

Trickett, Shirley, *Coping With Candida*, Sheldon Press, 1994

Virtue, Doreen, PhD, *Chakra Clearing: Awakening your spiritual power to know and heal*, Hay House, 2003

Walker, Morton and Shah, Hitendra, *Everything You Should Know About Chelation Therapy*, Keats Publishing, 1997

Waugh, Anne BSc (Hons) MSc CertEd SRN RNT ILTM and Grant, Allison, BSc PhD RGN, *Ross And Wilson Anatomy And Physiology In Health And Illness*, Churchill Livingstone, 2001

Weinberger, Stanley, CMT, *Candida Albicans: The quiet epidemic*, Healing Within Publishing, 1996

Wesselman, Hank, Ph D and Kuykendall, Jill, RPT, *Spirit Medicine: Healing in the sacred realms*, Hay House, 2004

Westcott, Patsy, *Thyroid Problems*, Thorsons Publishing, 1998

Williams, Xandria, *From Stress To Success: 10 steps to a relaxed and happy life*, Thorsons Publishing, 2001

Williams, Xandria, *Liver Detox Plan: The revolutionary way to cleanse and revive your body*, Vermilion, 1998

Wilson, James, ND, DC, PhD, *Adrenal Fatigue: The 21st Century Stress Syndrome*, Smart Publications, 2002

Windham, Bernard (ed.). Numerous research articles available at: www.flcv/dams

Woolger, Roger, PhD, *Healing Your Past Lives: Exploring the many lives of the soul*, Integrated CD Learning, 2004

Woolf, Victor, PhD, *The Wellness Manifesto*, The International Academy of Holodynamics, 2005. Available from: www.holodynamics.com

Ziff, Sam, Ziff, Michael, DDS and Hanson, Mats, PhD, *Dental Mercury Detox*, BioProbe Inc, 1997

Ziff, Sam, *The Toxic Time Bomb: Can the mercury in your dental fillings poison you?* Aurora Publishing, 1984

Useful Contacts

To find an amalgam-free dentist internationally:
International Association of Mercury-Free Dentists (IAMFD)
www.mercuryfreenow.com

International Academy of Oral Medicine and Toxicology
8297 Champions Gate Blvd
193 Champions Gate
FL 33896, USA
Telephone: +1 (863) 420-6373
Website: www.iaomt.org and www.iaomt.com

Holistic Dental Association
www.holisticdental.org

To find an amalgam-free dentist in the UK:
The British Homeopathic Dental Association
Menehey
Shawbury Lane
Shustoke
Coleshill
Birmingham B46 2LA
UK
Telephone: +44 (0) 16754 81535
Website: www.bhda.co.uk

The British Society for Mercury Free Dentistry
The Weathervane
22A Moorend Park Road
Cheltenham
Gloucestershire GL5 OJY
UK
Telephone: +44 (0) 1242 226 918
Website: www.mercuryfreedentistry.org

For information about holistic dentistry:
Dr Hal Huggins' clinic
www.hugginsappliedhealing.com

Dr Phillip Sukel's clinic
www.midwestdentistry.com

Dr Mark Breiner's clinic
www.wholebodydentistry.com

For information about electromagnetic pollution:
Powerwatch UK
Can assess electromagnetic pollution and sells devices
www.powerwatch.org.uk

American Society of Dowsers
Post Office Box 24
Danville
VT 05828
USA
www.dowsers.org

Canadian Society of Dowsers
www.canadiandowsers.org

Laboratories/tests:
www.genovadiagnostics.com

www.metametrix.com

www.doctorsdata.com

www.gdx.net

www.vrp.com

www.bodybalance.com

www.greatplainslaboratory.com

www.immuno-sci-lab.com

www.yorktest.com
(for food sensitivity blood tests)

www.melisa.org
(for MELISA test for hypersensitivity to
metals)

www.ccrlab.com
(For Clifford Materials Reactivity Test)

Information about mercury toxicity:
www.neuraltherapy.com and
www.klinghardtacademy.com
(For information by Dietrich Klinghardt)

Andrew Hall Cutler PhD PE
www.noamalgam.com

www.toxicteeth.org

www.mercurypolicy.org

www.angelakilmartin.com

www.momsagainstmercury.org

www.marytocco.com
(Mercury in vaccinations)

www.pamshelpline.com
Telephone: +44 (0) 1933 653339

www.flcv.com/dams
(For research articles on dental
amalgam)

www.lynrennickampssociety.co.uk

For supplies:
Wholistic Research Company
(healthy living products)
www.wholisticresearch.com

www.magneticclay.com
(For magnetic clay)

www.sekebal.com
(for SeKeBal Harmonie Gel)

www.surgeofchi.com
(for chi exercisers)

Tools for Energy, Balance & Health
25 Hainthorpe Road
London SE27 0PL
Telephone: +44 (0) 845 658 0012
Website: www.toolsforenergy.com
(For magnetic and other aids)

www.swissmasai.co.uk
(For information about Masai Barefoot
Technology trainers)

www.juliajohnson.co.uk

www.health-wise.eu
(For devices to combat electromagnetic
pollution)

For a practitioner:
Perrin Technique practitioners:
www.theperrinclinic.com

Nambudripad's Allergy Elimination
Technique practitioners (NAET):
www.naet.com

For a kinesiologist:
www.kinesiologyfederation.org

www.icakusa.com

www.kinesiology.net

International Association of Specialized
Kinesiolgists (ASK)
www.iask.org

Australian Kinesiology Association
P.O. Box 233 Kerrimuir
Melbourne
Victoria
Australia, 3128
Tel: +61 1300 780 381
www.kinesiology.org.au

New Zealand Touch for Health
Association
http://www.kinesiology.gen.nz

For a colonic hydrotherapist:
www.colonhealth.net/usa

Association and Register of Colon
   Hydrotherapists (ARCH)
Telephone: +44 (0) 1442 827687 or +44
   (0) 870 241 6567
Website: www.colonic-association.org

For information about Atlas Profilax:
www.atlasprofilax.ch

International Organisation of Atlas
   Profilax Professionals
www.atlasprofilax.org

Courses
For information about Touch for Health
   courses in the UK:
www.touchforhealth.co.uk

For information about Touch for Health
   courses in the US: www.tfhka.org
   (Touch for Health Kinesiology
   Association, USA)

For dowsing courses in the UK:
   www.britishdowsers.org (The British
   Society of Dowsers)

For dowsing courses in the US:
   www.dowsers.org (American Society
   of Dowsers)

Information about Fibromyalgia
National Fibromyalgia Association (US)
   Website: www.fmaware.org

Fibromyalgia Association UK
Website: www.fibromyalgia-
   associationuk.org

Information about CFS/ME
The National ME Centre
Old Harold Wood Hospital Site
Gubbins Lane
Harold Wood, Romford
Essex RM3 0AR
UK

Telephone: +44 (0) 1708 378050
Website: www.nmec.org.uk

Action for ME
PO Box 1304
Wells
Somerset
UK
Telephone: +44 (0) 1749 670799
Website: www.afme.org.uk

ME Association
4 Corringham Road
Stanford-le-Hope
Essex SS17 OAH
UK
Telephone: +44 (0) 1375 642 466/
   +44 (0) 1375 361 013 (Information
   line)
Website: www.meassociation.org.uk

ME Action
www.meactionuk.org.uk

For an informative site about CFS
www.drmyhill.co.uk

**For alternative information about
health**
www.mercola.com

www.wddty.com

**For video interviews about health and
consciousness:**
www.consciousmedianetwork.com

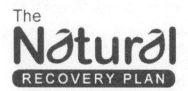

For support and community and to stay
up to date with all the latest information
on recovering from Fatigue Related
Syndromes visit the author's website at:
www.thenaturalrecoveryplan.com

Index